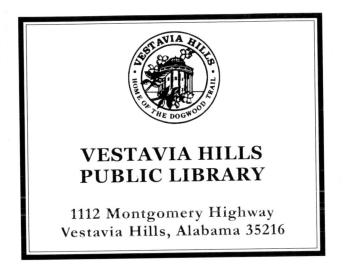

The Body Broken

The Body Broken

A MEMOIR

Lynne Greenberg

Random House | New York

Published in the United States by Random House,
an imprint of The Random House Publishing Group,
a division of Random House, Inc., New York.

RANDOM HOUSE and colophon are registered
trademarks of Random House, Inc.

Permission credits can be found beginning on page 217.

Library of Congress Cataloging-in-Publication Data
Greenberg, Lynne A.
    The body broken : a memoir / Lynne Greenberg.
        p. cm.
    Includes bibliographical references.
    ISBN 978-1-4000-6742-8
    1. Greenberg, Lynne A.—Health.   2. Chronic pain—Patients—
United States—Biography.   3. Neck—Wounds and injuries—
Patients—United States—Biography   4. College teachers—New York
(State)—New York—Biography   5. Chronic pain—Poetry.   I. Title.
    RB127.G743   2009
    616' .0472092—dc22
    [B]   2008023498

ISBN 978-1-4000-6742-8

Printed in the United States of America on acid-free paper

www.atrandom.com

9 8 7 6 5 4 3 2 1

First Edition

Book design by Adrianna Sutton

To Eric, Benjamin, and Lilly

The mind is its own place, and in itself
Can make a Heaven of Hell, a Hell of Heaven.
     —JOHN MILTON

Contents

PART II: A PARADISE WITHIN

EPILOGUE

Prologue

I was nineteen. Home from college for the summer. A third date. A reckless boy. I find myself initially unable to recall his name, having blocked it years ago—Walter, perhaps? My mother, emphatic, reminds that his name was Martin. All I remember is his stocky build and that, like a wrestler, his center hung low in his hips.

On our first date, we rode horseback. My horse bolted, and I fell. On our second date, he took me skeet shooting at his father's hunting club. The gun backfired, and I fell again. Shouldn't these falls have presaged another? Grounded, solid, he had a gravitational pull on me.

On our third date, we drove out from the suburbs of St. Louis, my hometown, to a friend's farm in rural Missouri. Huge party. Lots of beer stowed in his trunk, still unopened. He sped along faster and faster, eager for the fun to begin. Racing and bumping along the dirt road, the car hit a small ditch. Martin lost control of the wheel, and the car pitched, rolled, and tumbled off a thirty-foot drop. Those were the days before laws prescribed seat belts; none of us bothered to wear them. I flew out of the open window and fell, yet once more, landing in a cornfield far below. The car was totaled; people assumed that I was dead somewhere inside all of that bent metal. Martin suffered few injuries, a mere broken collarbone, and barreled out of the wreck.

I felt only a vague annoyance during the accident, at first, because hitting the ditch made me bungle my attempt to put on more lipstick. As we began catapulting off the embankment, I still felt no fear, anxiety, or even premonition, just more annoyance. This is so stupid, I thought. Now we're going to be late to the party. And then the sudden whoosh of being lifted high into the air, so brief this flight before the free fall, followed only by blackness.

News of the accident spread through the party. My neighbor Clayton Varley, hearing, raced to get to the car, taking a shortcut through a cornfield. He never found the car; he found me instead, lying among the ripening stalks. Dress ripped off. Unconscious. Covered in filth, rocks, glass, and blood. I was later told that he took his shirt off and covered my exposed body. Such a sensitive, protective gesture. One that sometimes creeps up on me unawares. I still find myself using it as a way of gauging individuals, particularly men. How would they behave in a moment of female vulnerability?

I came to in an ambulance, strapped to a gurney. I couldn't move. I could barely open my eyelids. They were swollen shut, but a man inches from my face demanded attention. He kept questioning me—my name, age, address, where I hurt. Again, I felt annoyance. I wanted to go back to sleep. My neck hurt. My arms hurt. My legs hurt. My face hurt. I answered a few of his questions but then drifted. Darkness again.

I awoke to a torture chamber of cures. A team of doctors was cleansing and stitching up my wounds. Screaming, I tried to writhe away from the several nurses who were holding me down. The doctors, waiting on X-ray results of my neck, would not give me pain medication, even a topical numbing agent, until they had identified my injuries. The doctors took for granted that I should endure my leg being sewn back together—the prick and then shudder of thread as it sliced through my skin—at the same time as they gouged pieces of glass out of my face and set my two shattered arms with no anesthesia, manipulating and yanking the bones into alignment. It was the night I first learned the many faces of pain, his different guises, sensations, and methods, and how clever he is at shape-shifting.

My mother reassured me that everything was going to be all right, but then I heard her sobbing outside in the hallway a few minutes later. The sound terrified me, but my mouth, too swollen and bruised, couldn't form the words to bring her back into the room.

Later that night, a doctor told me that my neck had been fractured. Without further explanation, he finally gave me pain relief—morphine—and for the next weeks in the hospital, time and consciousness bled. The days were sordid and vague. Constant pain. Constant nausea. The morphine made me throw up repeatedly, but, because I had to remain immobilized, I needed three nurses to do so. I would frantically press the call button, and nurses would rush into the room. Together, on a count of three, they would lift the sheet in one quick motion. My whole body would roll sideways so that I could reach the basin by my head.

Background noise during the first week of internal injuries, questions about future fertility, the risk of paralysis. Visitors punctuated the hours of unconsciousness. A Hallmark card arrived from Martin. "Get well soon!" it cheerfully announced. Noticeably absent were the words "I'm sorry," and in carefully crafted rhetoric, he denied any accountability for the accident.

Martin had been in the ambulance with me as we went to the hospital. Sitting on a cot above me, he had casually swung his feet too close to my body. I was going in and out of consciousness, but I remember clearly that foot of his. I worried that it would hit me in the face. He seemed oblivious to me and my injuries as he talked to the medic. I remember him wanting attention, babbling on about his shoulder. Ignoring Martin, the medic had knelt over me and eventually pulled a curtain across the ambulance to separate us. I never saw Martin again.

I underwent some kind of procedure for my neck fracture, but I'm not exactly clear when that occurred. I awoke to find my head no longer resting on the bed. I lifted one of my arms to try to feel why. My fingers met metal—a brace that encircled my head protruded about four inches from my skull. Further inspection of the contraption revealed that four holes had been bored into my skull and that the brace had been screwed into my head at these four sites. The device, called a halo brace, emphasizing the metal ring around my head, was held in place by a tight-fitting corset that encased my entire torso. I had metamorphosed into Frankenstein's monster.

Released from the hospital once I was stable, I spent the next two months recuperating at my parents' house. I didn't experience high levels of pain, mostly discomfort at having to wear the brace and a slight revulsion at having to clean around the four holes in my skull. My mother cared for me all summer to the point of exhaustion. Slivers of comfort, of sensory pleasure, came by way of food and music. My mother took to driving weekly to a bakery twenty minutes from our house to get my favorite cake—seven thin layers of yellow cake separated by fudge. Rather than regular icing, the entire cake was dipped in gooey chocolate. What had once been an annual birthday indulgence became my daily fare. I ate slice after slice at nearly every meal. I whiled away the days of boredom watching James Bond movies and Zeffirelli's *La Traviata*. My best friends Peggy Schmidt, Betsy Schechter, June Varley, and Miriam Tennenbaum came over regularly to keep me company in this period of enforced immobility. Listening to Rickie Lee Jones and Elvis Costello, we would chat about all of the typical things that college students on summer break discuss: their waitressing jobs, dates, parties, sunbathing at the public pool, diets, and more dates. I am ashamed to admit that I have lost touch with all of these women except for Betsy; mostly because when the halo brace came off, I barely set foot back in St. Louis again.

At the end of the summer, the doctors told me that I was something of a medical miracle. Apparently, this vertebra, the C2, is so high in the neck that it juts into the skull, nearly touching both the brain stem and the spinal cord. The bone, destabilized, usually slices one or both in half, causing, if not death, then permanent paralysis. It seems that only the barest percentage of people live (5 percent)—let alone walk (5 percent of the

5 percent)—after breaking this bone. Yet my neck had healed; I had full mobility and no other internal injuries of any consequence. I would be just fine.

Most of the adults in my life attributed my good fortune to divine intervention. In my jaded opinion, however, no greater spiritual source accounted for either the accident or my recovery. When various well-meaning friends of my parents sent me copies of Harold Kushner's now classic book *When Bad Things Happen to Good People* (if I remember correctly, I received five copies in all), rather than read it or glean any moral or religious lesson from my experience, I instead laughed in the face of larger meaning. My friends and I had a ritualistic bonfire in my wastebasket, burning every last one of the books. I was young, fearless.

I went back to college only two weeks late and spent the next three years making up for lost time—a little wilder, a little more eager to party, perhaps. I looked upon Brown University not as an academic institution but as one big playground. I spent the year dancing at weekly parties that my housemates and I threw—Rufus and Chaka Khan, the Talking Heads, and Marvin Gaye blasting into the wee hours.

I also took, in fact, no academic classes at all that year, only dance classes. Once upon a time, I had wanted to be a ballerina. So goes the story of countless little girls, I know, enchanted by the smell of the wood floors, the lyricism of the music, and even the attire—the second-skin leotards, pink tights, and satin toe shoes. I had commitment, anyway, taking dance classes nearly every day of my life since childhood. With my too-flat feet and too-wide hips, however, ballet was not a realistic career, and at nineteen I rarely considered whether I was good enough to dance other forms professionally, assuming that I would finish college first.

That car accident destroyed any chance I might have had of a later professional career as a dancer; my neck has never moved much since. Yet dance saved me after the car crash. A year of intensive dance classes, ballet, jazz, and modern, rather than physical therapy, repaired my body and spirit. I would carefully detach the neck collar which the doctors insisted that I wear for six months and, finally feeling like myself again, would spend hours at the barre pushing my body to regain its old flexibility and strength. One of the true beauties of Brown University's lack of distribution requirements is that a student can actually get away with taking only dance classes. The other beautiful thing about Brown—my appalled parents only discovered how I had spent the year (and their tuition money) well after classes had ended, when my report card arrived home. I did at least get straight A's that year. (I think it's hard not to get an A in a dance class, frankly.)

The car accident had unleashed chaos, but order had been quickly restored. The accident didn't change me—not in any profound way. Impervious to viewing the accident as life-altering, I experienced no startling or epiphanic insights. Nor did I develop any new ethos, worldview, or philosophy in the wake of the ordeal. The only psychological aftershock of the accident was that I became phobic of heights, mostly of falling. I wear the angry scars that run up and down my legs as my own red badge of courage, and I have hidden the permanent holes on either side of my temples with bangs for decades. I had neatly sidestepped death; walking away, I assumed, unscathed, I rarely thought about the accident again. In later years, the event merely served to confirm my status quo—decidedly fortunate, nurtured.

And alive.

PART I

Paradise Lost

. . . sights of woe,
Regions of sorrow, doleful shades, where peace
And rest can never dwell, hope never comes
That comes to all; but torture without end.
  —JOHN MILTON

CHAPTER I

A Wilderness of Sweets

A wilderness of sweets . . .
Wild above rule or art; enormous bliss.
   —JOHN MILTON, from *Paradise Lost*

I live on Garden Place in Brooklyn Heights, New York. A sleepy idyll, forgotten in the crazy speed and riot of New York City, it rests outside of time and outside of the cacophony. Only one block in length, the street is made up of single-family town houses and brownstones. Someone usually has to die for a house to go on sale here. Tree branches overhang the street, flowering pink puffballs of cherry blossom in springtime. They create canopies over the children, who are permitted to play ball in the street without supervision. On warm evenings, they gather for capture the flag, skateboarding, and manhunt, screaming "Car!" and racing to get out of the way of the occasional interruption. Everyone on the block dutifully shovels the snow within hours of a blizzard, puts out the trash only on designated garbage days, and responsibly accepts FedEx packages for the neighbors. People's window boxes change seasonally and predictably: mums in fall, evergreens in winter, daffodils in spring, geraniums in summer. If a baby wails late at night, a family goes on vacation, or a child gets into Harvard, the neighbors are the first to know. The street whispers safety, stability, understated affluence. There should be no failures on Garden Place or bankruptcies or terrors or tragedies.

We like to play dress-up at nightmare only. Every Halloween, the block becomes the center of such a maelstrom. It takes off its apron and goes all dark and wild—but only for the night. Unlike people in other parts of the neighborhood, we wait to

begin decorating our houses late that afternoon, as if to empha-
size that misrule and mayhem, evil and chaos, only occur for one
night here and will be exorcised by morning.

In a flurry of activity, we make over the street with only a few
hours to spare. The ornamentation is not elaborate; most of the
decorations were purchased a decade before and still retain a bit
of dust from having been hauled out of the basement. Glow-in-
the-dark skeletons hang in effigy out of second-story windows,
clumsily carved pumpkins line the stoops, and cobwebs festoon
the gates and trees. The homemade, somewhat tattered props
suit our block: they shroud it, offering just the right sprinkling
of decay and spook to transform the carefully maintained pret-
tiness of our street.

At five o'clock sharp, street traffic is prohibited, and we offi-
cially open our doors. Lugging baskets filled with candy outside,
every family on the block settles on the front stairs, adults with
cocktails, children with macaroni and cheese. My family—my
husband, Eric, and two children, Benjamin, fourteen, and Lilly,
eleven—always invites a crew of extended family and friends to
join us. My only rule is that everyone who comes over that night
should wear a costume. My love for my family rises exponentially every year as I see them struggle to comply with this rule.
My usually elegant brother-in-law Nick permits us to swathe
him in purple velvet swashbuckler attire. My mother-in-law,
Maria, unrecognizably silly, giggles in a clown costume, while my
refined sister Jeanne gets funky in a seventies rainbow-colored
Afro and platform shoes, and my brother-in-law David raps in a
blue polyester tuxedo and bling. My children's costumes, long
discussed, carefully conceived, have evolved in response to their
growing maturity: Tinker Bell transformed into a teenage rock
star; a dalmatian devolved into Dracula. I tend to like wearing
small touches only, usually accessories that somehow hint at my
mood that year: a black pointy witch's hat, crown, Mardi Gras
mask, fairy wings.

The crowds begin to pour onto our block. People from all

over Brooklyn gravitate to Garden Place, and it becomes one big street party, more and more raucous the later it gets. Our block plays the role of sentinel that evening. We are polite, even generous overseers of the madness, but always above the fray. The crowds of trick-or-treaters press, forming lines at the bottom of our stairs. We sit midway up our stoop, just high enough to make it difficult to reach us. In control, we casually toss candy from above into the up-stretched candy bags. "One piece per trick-or-treater only," we remind the younger helpers on our stairs, "or we'll run out!" Minutes later, we holler, "Friends always get extra candy, though," bending the rules for the familiar.

The evening will eventually teeter on the brink of sourness, as make-believe chaos gives way to potential threat. Dark descends and unruly teenagers wearing gas masks or burglar panty hose replace the toddlers dressed as princesses and firemen. A teenager leaps over a fence into the neighbors' yard to kick in a pumpkin and grab fistfuls of candy. Our block is momentarily shaken but reminds itself that this is only a night of pretend. All we have to do is stand up, brush the candy wrappers off of our costumes, and go inside, firmly closing the door to such nonsense. Danger, indeed—not on Garden Place!

When my family first moved onto the block, a neighbor told me how much candy to buy. I thought she was exaggerating—she wasn't. In those three hours, we give away more than three thousand pieces of candy. I won't pretend that I go to Costco or Walmart to buy cheap hard candy in bulk or go online to buy some healthy alternative to candy. My children and I instead go to the grocery store, and they get to pick out whatever kind of candy they want—usually bag upon bag of the most deliciously disgusting candy one can buy: Reese's Peanut Butter Cups, Milky Ways, and 3 Musketeers bars.

Later in the afternoon, we sit in the middle of our living room, ripping the bags open, the chemical fumes of processed chocolate wafting around us. The kids love to wrap their arms around and then dump the piles of candy into the baskets.

"We always have the best candy, don't you think, Mommy?" Lilly asked me wistfully three years ago. Seven at the time, all pinky-glowing skin and downy dimples, she sat on the floor up to her elbows in Hershey's Kisses.

I agreed with her. We did have the best candy. And, for some reason, that gave me immeasurable pleasure. Not because I was in competition with my neighbors, but because it somehow symbolized all of the particular sweetnesses of this period. And nothing made me feel safer than raising my children in this tiny enclave of Brooklyn. The neighborhood sang a tranquil lullaby that rocked any anxieties to sleep. Perhaps it is human nature not to remember that the simple line "rock-a-bye baby" is followed inexorably by "the cradle will fall." And even though so many of our nursery rhymes and lullabies describe this fall—when the bough breaks, when London Bridge fell down, when Humpty Dumpty took a great fall, when Jack fell down the hill—I had no sense of foreboding that I, too, would come tumbling after.

Our lives were simple, simply "enormous bliss." These words were written by John Milton to describe Adam and Eve's life in Eden before the fall from grace. The poem *Paradise Lost* has acted as a touchstone for me for years. It is Milton's masterpiece, an extended retelling of the story of Genesis—Adam and Eve's lives in the Garden of Eden, their temptation, fall from grace, and eventual punishment. In contrast to the story as narrated in the Bible, Milton lingered in Eden, that "wilderness of sweets," lavishly expanding the description of Adam and Eve's lives before the fall for thousands of lines of poetry, and I finally understand why: it was just too lovely there for him to leave.

And too lovely in my own paradise for me ever to want to leave. I cherished home as much for my children and husband as for myself. Our lovely house, part Edith Wharton age of elegance, part mold and sagging disarray, allows for privacy and a sense of community. We live vertically: a parlor and dining floor for everyone, the second floor for Eric and me, the third floor for the children, and an overgrown garden of ivy and peonies for our dog. If I peek out of my front door, I am surrounded by intimate friends and well-known acquaintances. I never have to worry about forgetting some seemingly innocuous but critical detail in the children's lives—a chorus rehearsal or parents' night at their school. I can count on my network of girlfriends to remind me. This intricate web of support, even in the years before I truly needed and relied on it, was one of the sweetnesses of my life that I most savored.

My marriage with Eric, buoyed by children and community, offers the central haven. Eric and I have been together for twenty-two years. We first met in college at Brown when I was twenty years old, only a year after the car accident. Together, we shared an ability to sidestep danger that seemed to set the pattern for our lives: hints of trouble transformed into fortuitous events.

Fortune trumped fate even at our first meeting, which took place during a hurricane, but one named Gloria, that managed to veer back into the ocean before doing any real damage and gloriously permitted us to meet. I was alone in the apartment that I shared with my friend Audrey, the top floor of a four-story apartment building filled with students. I had looked out of the window periodically during the day as the storm built. Students, taking advantage of the gale, were roller-skating, biking, and gliding on homemade rigs with sails. Storekeepers busily taped up their windows to protect against the potential force of the wind. I didn't think much of the storm; I had a paper due.

That evening, the storm grew wilder. My electricity went out. I hadn't bothered following the advice of local weathermen and had no candles or matches in the apartment readily available. Scrambling in the kitchen, trying to light a half-used candle with the stove, I heard a crash. Two of the windows in my living room had shattered. Taping up the windows had also seemed an unnecessary precaution. Regretting my earlier nonchalance, I raced out of the apartment and began knocking on doors.

After trying three floors of apartments without success, I finally found someone who was at home on the first floor. The young Eric, blond, thin, patrician, answered the door. He was holding a croquet mallet in his hand and waved me in. Candles lined the walls, illuminating an elaborate game of croquet and a bottle of champagne chilling in a bucket. There was no furniture in the room except for a plastic lawn table beneath an open sun umbrella and six chairs, remnants of a garage sale that for fifty dollars had allowed him to decorate his first apartment. I stayed that night until the storm was over, playing croquet, drinking champagne, watching card tricks, playing poker, staring into Eric's changeable blue-green eyes. I liked his calm. I liked his cool. I was smitten.

He was deciding. It took several weeks of awkward attempts at connection—an unexpected shortage of eggs, lost keys, could I borrow his phone—before he asked me out on our first date. Or was it a date? He wondered if I was hungry and wanted to get an ice cream with him.

We always joked in later years that he would tell me when he actually started liking me only on our wedding day. I would just have to wait until then for the mystery to be revealed. We knew for years that we would get married. My mother, so sure of this event, started planning the wedding a year before we actually got engaged. Thanksgiving 1990, she called me two days before we planned to come home for the holiday and informed me that we couldn't come. When asked why not, she admitted that it would be too embarrassing; everyone in St. Louis thought that we were engaged.

A college romance that could have ended in a broken heart, made worse by the public embarrassment of maternal expectation gone amok, instead ended in a marzipan rose of a wedding: pink rose centerpieces, rosebud boutonnieres, my dress bordered by satin roses. We married in my parents' backyard at sunset; it started to rain, but only after we had sat down to dinner under a tent. The downpour became just another symbol of our good luck. No one felt a drop. Eric's toast after dinner was a simple declarative—he had fallen in love with me at first sight and would love me until the day he died.

We howled with laughter later that night back in our hotel room, as he tried to get me out of the dress (an impossibility, really, with the two hundred tiny buttons down the back), while admitting that he had completely lied in the toast. He had started liking me about a week into my harassing him; he did consider the ice cream a real date.

The innocence of this first love left an indelible impression on our marriage, colored it magic, as if we managed to see everything in our lives, including the birth and raising of our children, through rose-tinted glasses. When I found out in my first pregnancy that I was having a boy, I was initially nervous. I was from a family of girls—what would I do with a boy? I began having anxiety dreams. A thick-necked hulk of a son would look at me, take a beer can, smash it on his forehead, and ask, "Yo, Ma! Wanna brewski?" Eric teases me that I made him read every line of the mother-to-be's bible, *What to Expect When You're Expecting.* We knew every small symptom, discomfort, and side effect of pregnancy intimately. We had complained about them together, each with a hand pressed to my belly, waiting for the next cascade of volcanic eruptions as our son moved or hiccuped. We felt ready. We were prepared. We had, however, not bothered to read that portion of the chapter on labor and delivery devoted to home birthing in case of a problem. As Eric pointed out, "Why bother reading it? What kinds of idiots don't make it to the hospital in time?"

So determined to experience the birth naturally, I stayed home with Eric for twenty-one hours as we took walks, warm showers, and listened to the Grateful Dead. When I was nearing pass-out, we finally decided that it might be a good idea to get to the hospital. We had miscalculated. We hadn't anticipated pouring rain, my not fitting into the backseat (Eric finally broke the front seat so that I could), traffic on the Brooklyn Bridge, no parking, a busy delivery room. By the time a doctor saw me, I was past the point of needing to push; the baby was "in distress." Distress gave way to miracle; Benjamin was born thirteen minutes later.

And that was thirteen years ago. Even the number 13 loses its cachet as unlucky in the context of our lives. The young man, Benjamin, captured at this moment, is another alchemy, dross turned into golden boy, mind all father, body all mother. His character comes from Eric: ebullient, enthusiastic, generous. He has what my family refers to as a "pure soul." If I am annoyed with him, he'll lean over to tell me that I'm the best mom in the world and then give me one of his goofiest, kindest grins.

He spends most of his time in motion: dancing, surfing, or skateboarding. When he was eight, on an August day, we had sat on the beach on Long Island looking at some boys about his age taking a surfing lesson. Benjamin wanted to try. Minutes later, I watched as an ecstatic Benjamin effortlessly stood up on the board on the first wave and rode it all the way in. "You killed it!" screamed his surf instructors. From that day on, Benjamin was theirs. Sunburst sea lions, they wrestle on the beach on days when the ocean is flat and "party wave," sharing rides, when the ocean swells. They also share lithe forms, agility, and a surprising grace on the water.

In their topsy-turvy world of speed, jumps, flips, and turns, to call something "dope," "sick," or "ill" is to bestow a compliment, to transform the appellation of misery into triumph. The irony of these misnomers did not resonate with me for a long time, probably because my own expectations about life were similarly unmindful of despair. I now watch shaken as Benjamin "cuts" waves, leaps in African dance classes, skis off picnic tables, and hurls himself down flights of stairs on his skateboard. My boy, the flier. And I keep whispering to myself, *Please, just let him keep soaring.*

In the early years of our marriage, Eric and my own flight seemed impervious to crashing. Even the heartache of a miscarriage after Benjamin's birth got assimilated physically. I barely had time to feel the weight of this bitterness as I got pregnant again three weeks later. Eric was out of town on the day of my scheduled sonogram. Benjamin, three at the time, towheaded, wild, and earnest, came with me to the appointment instead. We were both excited for him to meet his sibling. He sat perched at my feet as we peered at the monitor, both unsure of how to read the grainy images. When the doctor finished the measurements and confirmed that the baby was indeed healthy—and a girl—I got a little teary, only to erupt in laughter as Benjamin kicked me. Apparently, he had wanted a brother.

Lilly, the dulcet angel, was born in less than four hours of a labor untouched by drama or trauma. Her English teacher recently described Lilly as resembling one of the daughters in *Little Women*. "She looks like she should be coming to class in ringlets and a hoopskirt," he observed. She does have an old-fashioned beauty about her. With her midnight blue eyes, corn-flax blond hair, and fair complexion, she resembles her grandmother Maria who grew up in a little Alpine village in Switzerland. I sometimes think that we should have named her Heidi. Lilly also has the gentility and careful bearing of another era. I have watched so many adults try to connect with her only to find themselves stymied by her reticence. Once, we were introduced to a famous movie star, all extroverted glow and glare. He tried to charm her, telling amusing anecdotes in an increasingly animated fashion. She stared at him, placid, inscrutable, until he eventually gave up.

Yet while soft-spoken and reserved with adults, she is all giggles and chatter with her girlfriends. Her pack of friends has circled her around for years. In kindergarten, her friend Daisy stood at the classroom doorway nearly every morning waiting for Lilly. When Lilly would arrive, clinging to me, anxious, Daisy would grab her and pull her through the door into the classroom and, I always felt, into her life. Nowadays, the girls lock themselves in Lilly's room for hours without needing me or anyone else. Through the door, I hear snippets of conversation, laughing, the computer, music from *High School Musical*, the girls singing along.

For eleven years, raising Benjamin and Lilly provided the central rhythm of my life, one that generally permitted the private and public to coexist in harmony. My domestic, professional, and social worlds flowed together and in and out of each other. Before my children were born, this had not been the case. For a few years, my work had briefly demanded all of me. I had mistakenly wandered into a soul-killing career as a lawyer while in my twenties. I hadn't known what I wanted to do with my life, so my father had urged that law school would provide a "backup plan." I could "graduate last" in my class, if I wanted, "but just graduate." This career progressed in fits and starts without balance, and I fluctuated between intense periods of around-the-clock work as a lawyer and no work at all. These hiccups of on-again, off-again work culminated in my initially returning to work after Benjamin's birth but then lasting only three weeks at the job. I had a visceral reaction to leaving Benjamin; it felt untenable to continue working when at home nestled that soft, delicious bundle of a baby, and so I quit without discussion, planning, or thinking, this time for good.

Two years of full-time mothering ensued. Benjamin and I had an easy routine, our days structured by playgroup, music class, a nap, and the playground. Perfectly content to continue this lifestyle indefinitely, if our money didn't run out, I meandered into a poetry class on a whim—Dickinson, Yeats, and Auden—in the third year of mothering. I found what would prove to be my vocation. This audited class led to further literature classes, and as my passion grew, so, too, did the intensity of my studies. I worked harder than I ever had before, the drive and ambition fueled purely by love of the subject matter, and eventually completed a Ph.D. in English literature.

Always, I considered this degree a private pursuit. I had little expectation of getting a job as a college professor, knowing how hard these jobs are to come by. Most academics do not get jobs at all or get them in places in which they have no interest in living. Given Eric's work and our family life, I would not have the option of moving anywhere in the country to pursue my career. So when a job precisely in my field of interest (seventeenth-century British literature) opened up at Hunter College in New York City, a mere seven subway stops from my house, it seemed a chance for which not even I could hope.

I (miraculously, I always think) got the job, and, from the beginning, it permitted my life to remain balanced: the work challenging, even consuming, but not so all-consuming as to upset my domestic world. Hunter also allowed me substantial liberty to create courses that I wanted to teach and to control my teaching schedule. Teaching what makes me passionate inspired me and, I think, made me a more enthused teacher. Always in the classroom, I was aware of the luxury of getting to talk about what I loved with creative and engaged students. I also relished my scholarly writing—reading the latest criticism in my field and getting that spark of an idea that would evolve into a chapter or an essay. I particularly loved the academic conferences where we would spend the days listening to colleagues present papers and then stay up late over drinks, continuing the day's conversations.

My husband, too, after a record-breakingly short career as a corporate attorney, had found meaningful work as a journalist. For seventeen years, he has worked at ABC News. Beginning at the entry level as a desk assistant, he has now worked at nearly every conceivable job within the news division. A news junkie, he is never so happy as when a breaking story comes in from some far-flung spot, and he must race to get it on the air. His cool, the quality that most attracted me to him when we met, has also made him particularly good at handling the stresses of his work. During a "crash," he remains unruffled, logical, measured. I would find out only after my own crash how necessary this quality would come to be for our family. And to those who know him intimately, his equability translates into ethical compassion.

He is the first to offer aid, to come through for someone in need, or to show support. For me, he has always been the man most likely to cover and protect the body of a girl in danger.

I like to think that together Eric and I embrace the professions of both fact and fiction and that somehow this makes us whole. In the first thirteen years of our marriage, we were a two-headed Atlas holding up a world with a rich, full, and rewarding topography. We were living in the prime of our lives in our own little Eden. I was the luckiest girl in the world.

CHAPTER 2

Doom

Doom is dark and deeper than any sea-dingle.
—W. H. AUDEN, from "The Wanderer"

⁓ Twenty-two years after my car accident, in the last days of summer 2006, I sat nervously eyeing a physician's assistant. I had been walking around for weeks with head and neck pain, unable to move my head in any direction. Any movement or physical activity at all sent shock waves through the center of my head. I had treated these symptoms somewhat cavalierly at first, always assuming that my body would bounce back and that I would be fine, but my body had refused to do so. Staring at my MRI, the assistant finally announced, "Your neck is still broken." And in that breath of a moment, I could see that my life had fractured in two as clearly as had my fractured neck.

W. H. Auden ominously suggests that doom creeps up on the hapless and unsuspecting. Blissfully unaware, we suddenly find ourselves pitching out of our lives, tangled in the muck and weeds of fate gone awry. Upon the physician's assistant's pronouncement, down I tumbled and would drown in an abyss. I only questioned how I could have been so blind to the signs before now.

Milton, ever my inspiration, believed himself to be a prophet, in a lineage of blind seers like Tiresias who could divine the future. These prophets, associated with tragic stories, all foretold doom; I, conversely, had external sight but had had no premonition of a future of sorrow or pain. How was it possible that, after so many years of teaching Milton, I had not shared in or by osmosis learned the secrets of the oracle?

Perhaps we mortals see only what we want to see. I had simply ignored, evaded, and minimized the signs. There had been many. I had taken up jogging for the first time six months earlier, when a doctor had suggested it as a method of combating my early onset of osteopenia. How had I been oblivious of the dangers, when stories of running-related injuries are so rife? Running felt hard, punishing; it held none of the joy of dancing. I had relinquished physical pleasure. How could I be surprised that its antithesis would be the outcome?

There had been other foreshadowings of trouble as well. Eight years earlier, I had without warning permanently lost my sense of smell. I just suddenly couldn't smell anything at all. In an effort to reverse this loss, I had endured a painful surgery that opened up the pathway from my nose to my olfactory nerve. The surgery had proven ineffectual. Doctors could offer only hypotheses as to why—perhaps a virus, a rare side effect of pregnancy, or, more insidiously, a belated consequence of the head trauma I had suffered in the car accident. Similarly, only three years before, one of my wrists broken in the car accident had given out. At one of the sites of breakage, a large cyst had developed and was eating away the bone from the inside out. Another surgery. Another attempt to stave off wreckage. An X-ray of my other arm indicated the beginning of the same problem there (which would prove accurate, as it snapped a few months ago from a fairly minor fall). I was crumbling from within, my broken bones deteriorating over time. Why had it never occurred to any of us that my neck would be next?

The changes of the summer too should have forewarned doom. I had spent June and July of 2006 in London, doggedly trying to finish research on my next book, in which I had invested three years of research already. It was the hottest summer in England's recent history, and my work was grueling and solitary, punctuated only in the evenings by my children's stories of their many adventures with their babysitter, a London teenager whom we affectionately called Mary Poppins. While she led my children on excursions to museums, castles, plays, Renaissance fairs, street festivals, and parks, I enclosed myself in an un-air-conditioned, one-room archive in the House of Lords Record Office in order to slog through thousands of documents. For hours a day, I sat hunched low over nearly illegible seventeenth-century chicken scratch with a magnifying glass.

Two weeks into my work, I suddenly got a sharp, intense headache while working in the library. At first, I was so deep into the reading that I didn't notice it, but as the hours went by, it persisted. I had gotten to the library late that day and, focused on getting the work done, tried ignoring the pain, which didn't seem like it could be such a big deal. I had never experienced a headache intense enough to hinder my work before. My eyes started burning and tearing from the effort to read through the headache. I kept squinting to see better but found the letters blurring and nearly impossible to read. I finally had to stop working; frustrated, I vowed to get to work earlier the next day. In the morning, when I woke up, however, the headache was still there. It didn't go away, and it has never gone away since.

I first had my eyes examined, guessing that perhaps it was time for reading glasses, but my vision was normal. The headaches persisted and continued to get so in the way of my work that I visited a local internist. He concluded that these headaches did not fit the criteria for migraines and tentatively suggested that they might be tension related, brought on by the heat, stress of research, and living so far from home. Without doing a series of MRIs, however, he could not provide a better explanation of their cause. "No need for that," I reassured him, intent on not wasting any more days away from the library on such ridiculousness. My grant ran out in two months (as would my husband's patience at my having hijacked his children). The doctor accordingly prescribed some muscle relaxants and painkillers with codeine.

Though I was popping these pills constantly for the next six weeks, my productive periods became shorter and shorter, and I found myself having to prop books up on stands, because my neck also felt strained. I did still manage to finish the research on time and, relieved, returned to New York for a much-needed vacation on Long Island, where our family has gathered for years.

The headache continued unabated on vacation, however, and my neck became cricky, difficult to move, achy; still, I ignored these symptoms. Since the fall semester at Hunter begins the week before Labor Day, these last days before school were sacred rejuvenation and social time not to be interrupted by medical concerns. I luxuriated in dinners alone with my husband, candlelit hours of chatter on my sister's back porch, hours snuggling and reading with Lilly, and sunlit afternoons admiring Benjamin surf. I fondly remember the last time that I picked up anything of weight—my wiggling, giggling niece Coco. She was naked after swimming and wanted an ice cream. Wrapping her in a towel, I carried her from the beach. I remember thinking that her weight was straining my neck, but I brushed this thought aside, still feeling unbreakable and strong. No worries, as the Brits would say.

A few days later, I woke up unable to move my neck. Nothing unusual had happened the day before, just a particularly long run in the evening. Finally, belatedly worried, I sent out a slew of e-mails to friends and family, asking if they knew any neck specialists in New York. A neurosurgeon was highly recommended, and I drove into the city initially to see his physician's assistant. She ordered a series of MRIs and CAT scans and prescribed a strong anti-inflammatory and painkillers. I went back to Long Island, making a date with the local hospital to have these scans taken the Saturday of Labor Day weekend.

Unfortunately, I had to go back into New York City again two days later on the Friday of Labor Day weekend for my first day of work. My plan was to leave the family at the beach, take a bus into the city, teach, and then get the first available bus back to Long Island. I would even make it back in time for dinner. My

plan proved flawless, except for one problem. I found it difficult
to teach even the first, introductory classes (which usually consist
merely of handing out the syllabi, instructing students on my
house rules, and passionately riffing for a few minutes to get
them excited about the classes). I could barely carry all of the
Xeroxes. My head felt like it was caving in, and, unable to move
my neck, I had no peripheral vision to see most of the students
in the impossibly wide classroom. By the time I got off the bus
back on Long Island, I felt genuinely afraid. The pain was so
intense that I collapsed into the backseat of the car to lie down.
My husband drove us straight to my sister's home where the
whole family had gathered for a barbecue. In a state of physical
shock, my entire body violently shaking, I began to panic about
the intensity and speed of this breakdown. How would I teach?

Saturday's MRIs and CAT scans were a welcome relief. The
cold tunnel, the odd beeping noises, and instructions piped into
the tunnel all suggested the efficiency, certainty, and conclusive-
ness I had always associated with the field of medicine. I believed
that, unlike literary criticism, medicine did not have to contend
with metaphors with multivalent interpretations and associations. Doctors offered the surety of black-and-white truth. Just
the facts, ma'am. We were going to get to the bottom of this
problem and solve it pronto! On Tuesday, before I had to begin
teaching, I called the physician's assistant. She said that she had
received the radiologist's report of my scans, and although the
neurosurgeon was in surgery that day, she could meet with me
immediately. I would have my answer, solution, and a cure.

I never made it to Hunter that day—and I haven't been back
since. That morning in her office, the physician's assistant showed
me where a clean white line punctuated the black mass of the
bone in the scan. This line indicated that the base of that portion of the C_2 vertebra known as the dens was separated from its
top. The dens juts through the center of the C_1 vertebra and up
into the skull. At the apex of the neck, the dens should be a

lookout point, a watchtower standing guard over the brain stem, the main artery, and the spinal cord. It should rise strong and stable into the skull. Pointing to the expanse of white that sliced clean across the scan, she repeated, "Your broken dens never fused, do you see?"

CHAPTER 3

Falling

. . . I now must change
Those notes to tragic. . . .
    —JOHN MILTON, from *Paradise Lost*

꠸᪶᪶᪶ Peering at the scan, I nodded. Yes, I could see the break. Inwardly, I was still reeling from the news. For the last ten years, I had been absorbed by *Paradise Lost*, Milton's retelling of Genesis, of how the human race began; however, I had never bothered to ponder my own story of origins. Ironic, this lack of introspection. Perhaps, if I had been more self-aware, I would have realized even at nineteen that falling off a cliff was my genesis.

Two simple bites of an apple brought about Adam and Eve's fall—from grace, utopia, eternal life, joy, order, harmony, and peace—and the genesis of the human race. Not all falls have engendered such tragic narratives, and some falls have even been interpreted as triumphant. "Falling in love," in particular, describes one of humanity's most euphoric and sacred events, while "falling out of favor" signals the end of this privileged state. The fall of Icarus, his homemade wings a failure, emblematizes the defeat of mankind, but, then, Isaac Newton's dropped apple symbolizes man's resounding triumph. His discovery of gravity altogether reversed Icarus's fall, and human knowledge proved its mastery over the earth. Man had now reduced falling to a rational and logical scientific formula, seemingly stripped of the contours of tragedy.

Yet falling is tragic—to Adam and Eve and belatedly to me. My fall, a mere two seconds before landing in the sludge, dirt, and mire of a distinctly non-Edenic earth, unlike Adam and Eve's fall, was grand neither in scale nor in scope. An intensely private and individuated event, it managed only the minute consequence of beginning and now ending my former life.

I left the doctor's office with a follow-up appointment scheduled with the neurosurgeon but no other advice as to how to proceed. I was in a state of shock, beset by adrenaline and confusion, aware that my life had gone awry. I walked out into the busy New York street, and a person hurrying past knocked into me. I suddenly felt vulnerable, confused how, with a broken neck, I could be allowed to walk back out into the world. To do what? To go to Bed Bath & Beyond and buy a mirror, as I had originally planned, and then go teach all day? Was normal life supposed to continue? Or was I going to die? I felt prickly tingles at my fingertips. Was I losing feeling in my body? Was it spreading up my arms? Had the bone moved? Was I becoming paralyzed?

I was having a panic attack, I admit now, but I had never had one before. I didn't know how one felt. Can I at least blame the physical symptoms on my newly prescribed painkiller? Tingling at the nerve endings is one of its side effects. When I called the physician's assistant minutes after leaving her office and told her of my symptoms, she suggested that I head over to the emergency room at the hospital just as a precaution. Clutching the scans and reports, I rushed to the hospital's emergency room. When the waiting attendants heard my story, they placed me on a gurney and immobilized my neck. Memories of the car accident came surging back for the first time in more than twenty years.

The neurosurgeon, who had never even met me, had a break between surgeries and kindly saw me immediately. Upon looking at my films, he ordered more MRIs. More scans. Hours of waiting ensued. I began to call people on my cell phone, my arms the only part of my body that remained unfixed to the gurney. This hint of normalcy, making phone calls, distracted me from my panic, and soon I was joined by Eric and, later in the day, several members of my extended family, all offering moral support. My brother-in-law Marc, a Harvard-trained doctor and loyal to a fault, only left my side once that whole day—to join the radiologists who were reading my scans. Able to interpret the medical jargon, he could pronounce with as much certainty as the other doctors that my scans showed no indication that the still-broken C2 vertebra had become any less stable since the previous set of scans taken three days earlier. Further, they saw no indication of edema or bleeding that would suggest a new injury. My story—a summer of hunching over books and running—the neurosurgeon considered "soft." I had experienced no recent accident, no fall, no whiplash to account for this sudden onset of pain. Most reassuringly, in the doctor's opinion, I was not at imminent risk of paralysis and did not need spinal surgery to fuse the vertebra.

As suddenly as I had found myself strapped to the gurney, I found myself unstrapped and advised that I could go home. A traumatic day, but certainly not a tragic one. My fears lifted, although the cause and source of my pain remained unanswered, and Eric and I made our way home. In the months to come, as the cause and source of my pain continued to evade doctors, I would learn that medicine, contrary to what I had previously thought, is not a science of black-and-white facts but rather an art, capable of endless possibilities and as open ended as literary interpretation. I had never before fully embraced deconstructionist criticism. This technique consciously looks for inconsistencies and multiple meanings in a text, and I had always found it too nihilistic. In the field of medicine, however, I eventually became a confirmed deconstructionist. The multiplying and constantly shifting diagnoses offered by doctors lacked any stable meaning. Although doctors claimed to be interested in a logical narrative rather than a "soft" one to explain my pain, as the year progressed, the narrative arc of my story caved as surely as any deconstructionist would have predicted.

CHAPTER 4

Pain Diary

And so, from hour to hour, we ripe and ripe,
And then, from hour to hour, we rot and rot,
And thereby hangs a tale.
—WILLIAM SHAKESPEARE, from *As You Like It*

Once the neurosurgeon definitively announced that I didn't need surgery, I began visits to his pain management department for nonsurgical interventions to heal my neck and headache. Diagnoses proliferated, my "tale" boiling down to the rotting of old age—greater occipital neuralgia, cervical spondylosis, cervicalgia, degenerative disk disease of the cervical spine, arthritis, osteopenia, a bulging disk, a herniated disk, facet syndrome of the cervical spine, myofascial cervical pain, and new daily persistent headache. My neck had simply exploded under the pressure of so many overlapping problems. The old history of the unfused dens fracture lurked only as a subplot, a footnote initially in the prevailing diagnoses.

To address the many possible reasons for my pain, I spent September and October making weekly visits to the pain anesthesiologist's office where he proffered various prescriptions. I relied very sparingly on two painkillers, the opioid oxycodone for breakthrough pain and tramadol for everyday use (which my doctor assured me was less addictive). Fearful of dependency, I took these painkillers no more than twice a week. I had several other choices of medications to try anyway: anti-inflammatories, antiepileptic drugs that target nerve pain, muscle relaxants, and numbing pads to stick on my neck. Veritable drug cocktails. I became a bartender, shaking up exotic concoctions; however, I did so awkwardly. Lacking a degree in pharmacology, I found myself beset by technical questions: Should I try the tramadol now with an anti-inflammatory? Or should I go for the oxycodone and a muscle relaxant? If I take the oxycodone today, when it's only Monday, then what if I have a difficult week and can't take it again? So maybe I should hoard it for another time? Oh, it's only two o'clock. I took my first dose late today. So does that mean that I should wait to take my next dose?

Despite all of these guessing games, and my best attempts at mixing effective drug martinis, I also didn't feel any better. The pain did not ebb, and the several medications had dramatic side effects. One medication in particular, Lyrica, made me feel so dizzy and loopy that I found it difficult to stand up without a head rush. Hand flattened against the wall for balance, I would teeter across my bedroom. Getting to the telephone or turning off a light became a sinister jest, as I slammed—literally, not metaphorically—into walls several times a day while on this drug (as well as its companion drug, Neurontin, to which a new doctor switched me later in the year). Weathering all of these side effects proved useless, however, as none of these drugs ever noticeably helped my pain levels.

My doctor also sent me to physical therapy twice a week. My first physical therapist, a bald and disheveled man alone in his dingy office, used his hands to manipulate my neck to bring back more mobility, massage techniques to try to lessen some of the pain, and exercises that I was to practice several times a day at home. I initially threw myself into this new activity—so optimistic that I could heal my body again through exercise. Ever the good student, I diligently practiced his exercises five times a day. For six weeks I met with him twice a week; but one day, his massage sent me home in even worse pain, leading to a spike that lasted for three days.

Scared to let him lay hands on me again, I turned to a more sophisticated physical therapy program located in a busy hospital. The outpatient rehabilitation wing boasted several high-tech machines and contraptions but was also a typically overburdened department. I often found myself at the mercy of physical therapists who themselves were subjected to hectic schedules, unscheduled emergencies, and rotating shifts. Obliged to trust veritable strangers, none of whom ever learned much about my condition, I met with a revolving door of well-intentioned but uninvested therapists.

My new regimen employed radically different techniques from those of my first physical therapist—all more passive and geared toward pain reduction. The sessions began with acupuncture in both my feet and hands. The acupuncture made me feel nauseous, sweaty, and woozy, which the doctor considered "a good physiological response." Next, I had a hot compress placed on my neck, a TENS machine placed in different areas on my neck, a sonogram rubbed up and down my neck, followed finally by a cold compress. This passive approach, which didn't even require at-home exercises, I liked much better, for the obvious reason that it demanded absolutely nothing of me. After two months of trying this approach to no avail, however, I gave it up. It was a complete waste of time, and I continued to dislike acupuncture.

My pain doctor had other tricks up his sleeve. He began injecting my neck with various medications. Excessively conservative, he refused to inject more than one joint or nerve at a time (on only one side of my neck) and no more than once per week. Nevertheless, these shots quickly escalated in intensity and intrusiveness as my pain continued unabated: superficial trigger-point injections into the muscles (fifteen in all, which he did in only two sessions) led to an anti-inflammatory shot into the C2-C3 joint, followed by shots of short-acting numbing agents into various nerves (four in all). These nerve blocks were diagnostic and could provide only temporary relief (sometimes for only a few hours). I was to keep a "pain diary" for twenty-four hours after the shot to evaluate whether my pain ebbed at all. If so, then the doctor would know that he had found the correct nerve, and he could then "burn" it in a more permanent procedure (one whose effects would last perhaps a year, until the nerve regenerated itself).

These later shots were the most brutal, as he snaked needles closer and closer to my nerves using fluoroscopic guidance and my own responses of "Yes, that hurts more" to steer him. After one particularly bruising procedure that had gone on for well over fifteen minutes without any anesthesia (let alone any anti-anxiety medication, which, I discovered later, is routinely offered at most such pain management departments), I turned to the doctor and said, "You know, we used to call you Dr. Pain at home, but now I think I'm going to call you Freddy—you know, from *Nightmare on Elm Street?*" His gathered staff tellingly all laughed outright.

Based on the results of these forays into my nerves, he diagnosed my primary problem as greater occipital neuralgia and thought the right occipital nerve a good candidate for burning. The burning procedure (again conducted with no medication) consisted of his sticking a needle into my neck for five minutes as he slowly blocked the nerve with phenol. He then left the needle dangling out of my neck, bopping into my range of vision, as he actually had the gall to leave the room. The needle, he explained, had to stay in my neck while the wound cauterized for another five minutes, so, not bothering to stick around, he said that he would be back when it was time to take it out. Even my rock-solid husband blanched. He had been seated next to me during the whole procedure while I gripped his hand. The needle now hung directly in front of his nose.

Neither that nor any future injection helped to reduce my pain, and I look back on myself in the early months of the fall as naïve. I submitted willingly, ever hopefully, to the shots, as I kept assuming that the next one would bring the relief I needed.

I could then effortlessly go back to my life. Preparing myself for each shot, I would reason that, while painful, it was worth it, if it could stop my pain. My attitude was akin to the overly simplistic adage "No pain, no gain." I didn't initially feel traumatized from the shots, as they were advertised as curative. The cure soon proved as cruel as the pain itself, however, and the repeated shots into my nerves left me exhausted, bruised, and disheartened. I would hobble into bed after each shot and spend the rest of the day on my side with an ice pack on the place he had injected. I also found that I was losing weight—at least two pounds after each such procedure. It was only after six of the nerve shots that I found myself thoroughly disgusted with and even phobic of the shots, primarily because they brought me no relief.

The doctor responded by suggesting that he inject one nerve at a time with the diagnostic block, moving all the way down my neck, nerve by nerve, until he found the correct one. A hit-or-miss approach, if ever I had heard of one, and a process that, at the slow rate he went, would take several weeks to accomplish. The most troublesome part of this plan, however, was that he definitively stated that it was too dangerous to inject the C2 nerve, even though we all knew that the big skeletal problem resided there. He wanted to begin instead to move in precisely the opposite direction, working his way down the neck from C4 instead. That was when I finally went looking for a new doctor.

My one regret is that I hadn't trusted my instincts better and searched for a new pain management doctor earlier. As the year progressed, I found that choosing the correct caregiver became a critical component of my healing process. "Not all doctors are healers," mused my friend Leslie, and I thought about how so many of my doctors that first year shared patterns of professional dispassion and scientific detachment that only masked dyspathy. Compassion, perhaps, was the foremost quality I needed from a doctor in the face of pain that had left me feeling so vulnerable. My father-in-law, Mike, a renowned nephrologist, had given me this advice early on: "Treat your injury as you would a research paper. Speak to as many people as you possibly can. You will undoubtedly learn something new from each of them. It will also give you the opportunity to 'interview' these doctors until you find the one you like the best." I only wish that I had listened to him sooner.

CHAPTER 5

A Broken Home

*In the heart of pain where mind is broken
and consumed by body, I sit. . . .*
—ADRIENNE RICH, from "1941"

It was now late fall in New York, and I had spent the last two months in a haze of shots and preoccupying pain. It seemed that every day, at some point, the pain would increase exponentially, bringing me to my knees. These pain spikes made life unbearable; and I found myself obsessed with guarding against them. Maternal abdication ensued.

Our domestic routines had functioned well for years. Benjamin and Lilly both attended school full-time and had a host of after-school activities all within walking distance of our house. Benjamin had long walked everywhere with friends or on his own, but Lilly still needed someone to shuttle her from one activity to the next. Because I went into Hunter three days a week, our long-standing babysitter Cora always dropped off and picked up Lilly on those days. The other two days a week, I took Lilly to her activities.

The first change in our daily routine was that I could neither pick Lilly up from school nor take her anywhere. Walking always seemed to exacerbate the pain, and I took to avoiding doing so. As the week progressed, the five city blocks to her school began to feel insurmountable. In the early fall, when I first found myself incapacitated, I logically assumed that my injury would heal quickly, so I turned gratefully to my close-knit group of neighborhood friends who mobilized with offers to pick Lilly up after school. When the days stretched into weeks, and I could still not resume my normal responsibilities, I realized that the makeshift help with Lilly would need to be more certain. I didn't want to burden my endlessly generous friends further and began to rely more heavily on Cora for round-the-clock help.

This relinquishing of control had several collateral effects—both financial and emotional. I justified the extra expense by assuring myself that the situation was only temporary. The strain on our finances did not initially overwhelm; it would take several months for this to occur, as my sick leave became unpaid and the doctors' bills not fully covered by medical insurance mounted. The emotional ramifications of relying so much on Cora shifted almost schizophrenically from one day to the next. I vacillated between gratitude, relief, guilt, and frustration, knowing all the time that I had no real choice.

Worse was the effect of my incapacitation on my relationship with Lilly. While seemingly perfunctory, our walks, so filled with chatter and the news of the day, had always functioned as important bonding time. Without this ritual, our relationship slipped just that little bit. I no longer had as close a handle on the daily nuances, her subtle shifts of emotion, or negotiations with the outside world.

Performing domestic errands devolved as my condition failed to improve. For a while I managed to accomplish errands like picking up the dry cleaning in a haphazard way, but grocery shopping was simply impossible for me. We initially made do with last-minute runs to the small grocery just around the corner. Eventually, Cora took over the grocery shopping as well. My former attempts at cooking (never much of a priority anyway) wholly dissipated. We did a brisk business with the neighborhood restaurants that delivered, and Lilly and Benjamin ate endless meals of pizza and Chinese food. They ate alone on too many nights, since, as the fall progressed, I roused myself out of bed to eat dinner with them less and less frequently. On the rare occasions when I did join the kids for dinner, my attempts at discussion were routinely greeted with hostility or, worse, intense sibling rivalry, as they competed for this tiny sliver of maternal attention.

I originally misinterpreted this change in their relationship. Benjamin had always been an ideal big brother; now he got annoyed at everything Lilly said at the table. Less patient with each other, they began to bicker. I attributed the strains in their relationship to the age difference, the onset of puberty, or exhaustion from such long school days. I went so far as secretly to applaud Lilly's growing assertiveness. Pat explanations all, glossing over problems. I had neither the stamina nor insight to question these initial conclusions, and it would take months to recognize that my injury had created tensions and anxieties in my children. These fears needed an outlet, and it was far safer to pick on each other than to turn on me—at least at first.

In the past, I had also been able to meet the children's material needs. There had always seemed to be a list of items to purchase, like new sheet music for the piano or larger sizes of socks, and endless activities to orchestrate—sleepovers, parties, and dance, piano, and tennis lessons. Like all working parents, I had kept detailed lists and juggled these responsibilities with my work, slipping in domestic phone calls between my classes or rushing to buy some item before jumping on the subway home. Prosaic, these efforts, but as the tasks became more unrealistic for me to accomplish, I realized how much my kids had internalized having their little needs met. My mundane efforts had provided a security blanket that tacitly assured them that someone was caring for and about them.

Subtle, at first, the way the kids responded to apparent neglect. Benjamin used my failures as an excuse to gain more independence. Before dinner, often when it was already dark outside, he would rush into my room and ask whether he could jump on his skateboard to go to Gamestop, as he didn't have a present yet for so-and-so's birthday. The rule had always been no going out alone once it got dark. Now on occasion I found myself bending that rule—the errand had to be accomplished, I reasoned, and I didn't have the strength to do it.

Lilly's response was more complex. In the late fall, I thought that Lilly had begun to show glimmers of stress. Perhaps in response to my condition and her anxiety over it, she seemed to be acting like a hypochondriac. After a few weeks of listening with increasing concern as she described nearly daily visits to the nurse's office, I called the head of her school. I worried that Lilly had inappropriately learned by my example that the way to get attention was to be sick or injured. After observing her for a few days, the head of the school called back to report that Lilly was just fine, "bubbly at lunch with her friends, sparkly even" at school. Nevertheless, at home she continued to use the excuse of a small cut, bruise, or runny nose to pile into bed with me. The extra cuddling and nurturing became for a while the easiest way for me to remain connected to her.

Eric and I worked hard to insulate both kids from the worst of my condition. I tried not to cry around them or let them see me when I was in the midst of a bad pain spike. Nevertheless, they were privy to far too much information. Concerned family members felt the need to check in daily. Perversely, this always seemed to occur when I was trying to focus on Lilly, reading with her or helping her with her homework. When a conversation became noticeably serious, I would refrain from continuing it in front of Lilly or Benjamin, yet far too often they overheard frightening news. In the early days of confusion and terror, Lilly once overheard me discuss paralysis with a doctor on the telephone. There might have been other such incidents; I honestly don't know.

Processing snippets was not all that was required of them during this period. When Lilly came home from school, she had always run up the stairs to burst into my room. That fall, whenever she did so, she invariably woke me up from a nap. I now implemented a new rule. No more open-door policy. If I was in my room with the door closed, then the kids were not permitted to enter. They were no longer welcome. Mama had slipped and, like Alice in Wonderland, was sliding farther and farther away from them, down the rabbit hole. I just couldn't figure out how to stop tumbling.

CHAPTER 6

Burning Nerves

The pain we feel reading
mere words in a book
clings to us like static
on a cold day. The road
a woman walks in the last chapter
twists away from her happiness,
and the pain follows
wherever we go, haunting us
with its mute footsteps—the ghost
of pain we have known

and of pain to come.
Small explosions
of grief in a sonnet sequence;
another fracture of innocence:
these are templates into which our lives
must fit themselves, moving shadows
the sun makes, rising and going down
on every page, as evening settles
into all the unswept corners
of the world.
    —LINDA PASTAN, "The Art of Pain"

By December, I barely got out of bed at all. I had come to the point where I found it easier just to lie immobile than to try to walk around or move, as physical activity always increased the pain. I rarely left the house, except to go to the doctor for shots. I had evolved, without clearly realizing it, into an invalid, lying prone with a long thin pillow slid under my neck, my bedside table laden with bottles upon bottles of pills.

I had always subscribed to the philosophy that you are what you do. Yet I no longer did anything. The activities of the healthy had no relationship to my diurnal existence. "What are you doing today?" someone would ask. How was I to answer this question? *I'm doing pain right now?*

Pain penetrated every mite of concentration, infiltrating in a full-frontal attack, a D-day to the body. It left me lethargic, dolorous; all I wanted to do was lie there. I was so preoccupied by my body beached that I allowed my mind to become a desert as well. I spent whole mornings just looking up at the graying white paint of my ceiling. If I rolled onto my side, then I could at least stare at the pale lilac walls or the drawing of the ballerinas that hung over the fireplace, but I didn't concentrate on this view: all thought monomaniacally revolved around my physical condition.

Benjamin, bubbling with excitement, interrupted one such wasted day. Bursting into my room where, as usual, I was lying flat on my back, he presented me with several odes he had written especially for and of me, and I saw that he was offering me what he thought would most please me. Unself-consciously, he read ode after ode that boiled down in subject matter to "Mom, I really love you!" With a flourish, he hushed my enthusiastic applause and announced that he had yet to read his greatest triumph, accomplished in his poetry class just that week—a sestina.

How complicated it is to write a sestina; the most intricate and elaborate of forms, it requires technical feats and immeasurable control to pull off: six stanzas, each six lines in length, and a final three-line terminal stanza. One is limited to the constant repetition of the same six words placed at the end of each stanza, and all six words must appear in the final three lines in a prescribed, precise order. The troubadours in the twelfth century developed this form, singing them for the entertainment of the French court, all trying to outwit each other by the versatility and complexity of their poems. Benjamin, with an enormous grin, blithely read me his perfectly conceived sestina, which unsurprisingly revolved around a surfing experience.

I gazed in admiration at Benjamin with his long, blond surfer hair askew, his still-tan skin shimmering. I adore my son, I thought. He has so fortunately inherited his father's love of hype, of outrageously exaggerated acts of unselfish, sheer spoiling. The puppy dog approach to showing love—larger-than-life expressions of loyalty, slobbery, unadulterated adoration, and pure whimsy.

His poem also inspired me; for the first time in months, I thought about writing, wondering whether I would be able to write a sestina. And so was born my idea of writing a volume of poetry—for once, no longer the critic, I would create an "art of pain," in the contemporary poet Linda Pastan's words; poetic forms would provide the "templates" into which I would fit the last few months of torture. I would call the volume *Burning Nerves*. Clever, I thought, oh so clever, as both words worked as puns to describe my experience.

I began with initial passion to work on this book, scribbling half-finished poems into a spiral notebook while still lying flat on my back in bed. The pen upside down, kept running out of ink; I switched to a pencil. My arms got tired, holding up the notebook for so long; I switched to a smaller notepad. Eager to feel useful and creative, I kept writing. Half-baked puns abounded. I was not the patient patient, but rather an impatient patient who should be an inpatient. Just because I was an invalid did not mean that I was invalid. My bone had refused to re-fuse. I was unnerved, so please unnerve me, doctor; my nerve pain was too nerve-racking, too enervating; my nerves had some nerve—frankly, they were a pain in the neck.

My "Ode to Oxycodone" (my current medication) inspired, or mutated, into a diptych, the companion poem prominently featured a skull. An epic derailed: "Neither of arms nor the man, I sing / Muse, do not talk to me of love and war / This life, shrunk to the size of my bed, / is no epic." I wrote a blazon, but rather than describing each idealized physical attribute of a lover ("her cheeks are like roses, her eyes as blue as the morning sky," and so on), I anatomized the internal horrors of my neck and head. Physical pain met psychological pain in one macabre sonnet. My body became Laura, the missing mistress of Petrarch's sonnets: "If I submit and silence myself too, / doctor, will you fix me? Make me whole again." An ekphrastic poem became a still life—so still was my life now. Trying a villanelle, I floundered just trying to come up with the necessary rhyming words. Nerve and perve? Phenol and fetal? Ablation—operation, obliteration? I eventually settled on pain, wane, feign, refrain, deign, and vain for the first set of rhyming words, but that was as far as I got. Finally, I attempted the beloved sestina, but it degenerated into an unfinished square dance with a sadistic ringmaster ordering me to do-si-do with my pain. No elegant court music or sophisticated wit here, just the country music of my Missouri childhood.

Poetic forms, the very architecture of my professional life, seemed to be crumbling all around me. Pain, I realized, does not fit into the tamed heartbeat of iambic pentameter. It pummels through borders. Unremitting, it refuses closure and explodes rhyme and reason. All-consuming, it does not permit the luxury of metaphoric or chiasmic thinking, tropes or symbols, wit or pun. Its sound is unsound, dysphony, a wail, silence. My "art of pain" was an artless descent into chaos, an all-too-perfect emblem for my life. There were no poetic words for this pain, just my racked body to signify it.

CHAPTER 7

Descent into the Underworld

Undone Persephone . . .
Uncomforted for home, uncomforted. . . .
    —EDNA ST. VINCENT MILLAY, from "Ode to Silence"

Only a few weeks before my life fell apart in 2006, Lilly and I spent our last day in London at the Tate. We wandered through the museum, chatting, looking, and enjoying one of the few oases of air-conditioning in the city. It was a scorcher outside, and, reluctant to face the heat again, we lingered for hours over several paintings. One portrait, in particular, mesmerized Lilly. By Dante Gabriel Rossetti, the painting is a portrait of Persephone. Looking strangely pale and unworldly, Persephone holds a crimson pomegranate, the forbidden fruit that would be her undoing.

The Greek myth of Persephone offers an explanation for the origin of the seasons. Hades, god of the underworld, sees the young maiden Persephone gathering flowers, abducts the unwilling girl and drags her down to the underworld as his bride. Grief-stricken Demeter, mother of Persephone and goddess of the harvest, begs Zeus for her daughter's return, threatening to keep the earth in perpetual barrenness unless Hades releases Persephone. Zeus agrees to do so, but only if she has not eaten anything in the underworld. Unfortunately, Hades had already tricked Persephone into tasting a pomegranate's seeds, a symbol of the consummation of their marriage, thereby binding her irrevocably to him. Zeus comes up with a compromise, permitting Persephone to return to earth and her mother for part of the year, but requiring Persephone to spend the other part of the year with Hades, as his queen. Demeter mourns during the months when her daughter is trapped in the underworld, which explains the harsh, cold season of winter. When Persephone returns, joyful Demeter blooms again, giving rise to spring.

I am haunted by the memory of Lilly and me standing in front of that portrait. That day at the Tate, Lilly and I had fixated on the painting, partially because she knew the myth from school that year and partially because the realism of the painting had captivated us. Rossetti rendered Persephone in great detail, and the expression on her face is so specific and complex as to somehow capture the many emotional shifts and changes of both her present and future—her initial unawareness, later confusion, and eventual sadness. On a personal level, the portrait gestures to my own predicament. That summer sojourn at the Tate freezes the period right before I lost my world, the same way the painting illustrates that moment for Persephone. And, like the story of Adam and Eve, Persephone's fate seems to parallel mine. Another story of origins, a fall, and the loss of earth.

I have always turned to literature as a lens through which to understand and interpret my life and to find the words to describe what has seemed ineffable in it. Now I relied on this familiar support, finding a literary analogue that put my situation into a new perspective. This painting seemed to prefigure my future, and I personalized Persephone's unique fall from grace. In *Averno*, a volume of poems that reinterprets the myth, Louise Glück describes Persephone's return to earth after her first descent into the underworld:

> As is well known, the return of the beloved
> does not correct
> the loss of the beloved: Persephone
> returns home
> stained with red juice. . . .

("Persephone the Wanderer")

I find this detail compelling; Persephone's and my mouth become one, bloodied from the juice of the pomegranate, from the loss of innocence, from the violence and pain wreaked on our bodies. And, like Persephone, I was entering my first winter in the underworld.

CHAPTER 8

Anxiety

Tell me this is the future,
I won't believe you.
Tell me I'm living,
I won't believe you.
—Louise Glück, from "October"

⟶ As the weeks stretched into months, I found myself bemoaning my nonlife, and I began looking at each subsequent doctor with increasing dread. Did I still belong to earth, or was I in hell? Would I, like Persephone, have to endure this shadow existence, ostensibly dead but perversely still alive, indefinitely? Or would I remain in limbo only temporarily? Please tell me that this isn't permanent. Please tell me that you can fix me.

Doctors, willing to try, repeatedly asked me for detailed accounts of my pain in the months to come, and I realized the importance of my descriptions for the diagnosis and cause of my pain, which still had no definitive explanation. While I would never finish my poetry volume, my aborted effort had helped me to acquire a vocabulary by which to explain my pain. I could with far greater accuracy and precision tell doctors where and how I hurt. I even had a legion of carefully crafted, nearly scientific narratives to explain my condition:

I am in pain from the moment I wake up until the moment I go to sleep. On a scale of 1 to 5, my pain never falls below a 3 and will rise at some point to a 5 nearly daily and stay there for hours. These spikes are unrelenting, stare-at-the-ceiling, wait-it-out pain. Its sinews unfurling, the pain whips through the middle of my head. It feels like an ice-cream headache—the sharp deep freeze of eating or drinking too much of a cold substance too quickly. It is heavier than an ice-cream headache, though; it feels as if an enormous weight lies along the tendon, crushing this central route, tearing my head in half. When spiking, the pain radiates out from the center and disperses. The ice cream has melted, not just freezing my forehead but dripping down to encompass my entire head symmetrically, pooling finally behind my eyes. Sometimes the pain is so intense that even the skin on my face, particularly around the eyes, hurts like a bruise. My eyes also burn and smart and sting. I would later learn that in scientific terms, one could describe my pain even more accurately as "retro-orbital," "holocranic," "halocephalic." In more emotional terms: Inescapable. Disabling. Punishing. Grueling.

These descriptions proved critical that winter. After the disastrous two months of shots administered by Freddy, truth, in the guise of a diagnosis, cure, and certain prognosis, became my personal Holy Grail; my family and I became thoroughly absorbed in the process of finding a new doctor. Daily calls and e-mails from family and friends recommended new neurosurgeons, pain anesthesia doctors, sports medicine doctors, craniosacral osteopaths, neurologists, endocrinologists, chiropractors, internists, kinesiologists. Sorting through the sheer number of possible specialists on whom to rely was in itself a full-time job, as I was often unclear as to which branch of medicine to turn. In order to try anything I could to get better, I visited several specialists throughout the months of November and December. These trips from Brooklyn into Manhattan became my career. They were, unfortunately, expensive, painful, and too often useless. The bumpy cab rides, ten times the cost of taking the subway (another daily activity no longer tenable), nearly always spiked the pain, and the appointments themselves were generally for naught.

Sometimes, though, they were harrowing. More than one doctor told me that I would never get better, and that my condition would only worsen as my body continued to age. One supremely unsympathetic neurologist, a self-proclaimed headache specialist, shook her head sadly, repeatedly proclaiming, "You have daily chronic headache. Very, very difficult to cure, you know. You really have to want to get better." I left thinking that I had caused a hopeless situation by not trying hard enough to improve. Another neurologist, in contrast, discounted my pain and concluded that nothing seriously ailed me. I just had a simple case of temporomandibular joint (TMJ) syndrome. Get a tooth mold and get out of bed.

I kept searching for answers, confused, frustrated, but altogether convinced that if I just found the right doctor, the right treatment, I could be cured. Another neurosurgeon announced that I had not been adequately evaluated for bone instability at C2. Only by having an MRI taken with my neck in positions of movement—looking up and down—could one determine precisely the attendant risks associated with the nonfusion. This threw me into a renewed state of anxiety. Three months had already gone by, and now I found that the proper scans had not even been conducted.

For a week I waited, fretting, preoccupied. When the MRIs finally came back, they only increased my fears. The bone was unstable. When I moved my neck, the bone at the place of the nonunion would separate, and each half would move in a different direction. The risk with such instability is that the bone, moving the wrong way, will sever the spinal cord or pierce the brain stem. The neurosurgeon assuaged my worst anxieties, discounting this risk, as the bone did not in fact touch the spinal cord when in motion. In his opinion, the amount of movement—three millimeters—did not constitute an imminent threat. Moreover, he wasn't sure whether this nonfusion was the real source and cause of my pain; he therefore advised that I should avoid surgery to fix the instability until I had ruled out every other possible reason for the cause of my pain, and he sent me back to the pain anesthesiologists.

In the meantime, my body continued to weaken. A visit to the dentist revealed that two of my back molars had split in half. My gynecologist found a lump in my breast (benign, it turned out). A new bone density test indicated that I had lost more bone mass. New X-rays of my neck suggested that the osteopenia in my neck had worsened. My weight continued to plummet. Blood tests revealed severe vitamin deficiencies. I interpreted all of these results as a further consequence of my neck pain; my entire immune system had begun to devolve in the wake of pain.

CHAPTER 9

The Loss of Language

I felt a cleavage in my mind
  As if my brain had split;
I tried to match it, seam by seam,
  But could not make them fit.

The thought behind I strove to join
  Unto the thought before,
But sequence ravelled out of reach
  Like balls upon the floor.
  —EMILY DICKINSON, No. 106

After so many doctors' appointments, I had developed a concise narrative to explain my condition and reason for making the appointment. I behaved at these meetings fairly rationally; I sounded intelligent, even articulate. Aside from my well-rehearsed descriptions of my medical condition, however, all logic seemed to have fled and language to have abandoned me. Not just one thought, as in Dickinson's poem, but all my thoughts and their "sequence[s] ravelled out of reach." In conversations with friends, I knew that I was repeating myself, forgetting basic vocabulary and names, sometimes losing the trail of the conversation, but I was incapable of avoiding doing so. I conflated incidents, individuals, events. In my opinion, literally because "my brain had split" from the rest of my body, I began to experience memory and language lapses. I knew that the medications were not helping my mental acuity either. Loopy and drugged out, I sounded as incoherent as I felt.

Words had always provided me with the sustenance that had given me intellectual and emotional stability for the past fifteen years. As the year progressed, I found myself unable to write a sentence or to read. At the time, I attributed this inability to my pain levels. How could one perform an act that requires mental concentration when one had the biggest headache of one's life?

My friend Susan suggested that I at least listen to books-on-tape and bought me several of them as a present (my favorite choice was Nora Ephron's *I Feel Bad About My Neck*). I listened to about four of these tapes, but all of that concentration needed to follow the stories gave me a bigger headache. Another friend suggested a Dictaphone with which I could at least record what I was feeling. It lay unused on my bedside table. Eric even bought voice recognition software for the computer, hoping that it would inspire me to write. I didn't turn on my computer for the next six months.

I had always loved sharing my passion for reading with my children. Benjamin had long read to himself, no longer needing my encouragement or involvement; Lilly still read aloud to me. Curled into bed together, we continued our nightly ritual of reading together, but I no longer followed the stories. Her words would dissolve into dust mites, fragments of sound. No more laughing and crying together over the details of the storylines, explaining difficult words to her or making sure that she understood complicated twists in the plots. Had we stepped through the wardrobe in *The Chronicles of Narnia* or been sucked into the tornado in *The Wizard of Oz*? I couldn't remember even what story we were reading, let alone its narrative.

Two events in particular emblematized for me the morbidity of my new existence, suffering from some form of aphasia. The first came when my colleague Michael's novel came out. He and I had discussed his work often. He had written a modern-day epic, the genre I most loved to teach. Having promptly bought Michael's book the moment it came out, I found myself staring at the first page—frustrated and confused as the words melded into an incomprehensible jumble. The pain in my head was so juicy, so fiery, that day that I simply couldn't read.

This had been happening for months. Important new Milton criticism would arrive, often a gift from the author. Remaining unopened, these tomes began to grow into piles, makeshift coffee tables in my library. I was exhausted just trying to read the introductions. My mind would twirl, the sentences would blur into gibberish, and I would put the book down, deflated, and begin staring up at the ceiling again. "I can connect / Nothing with nothing" (T. S. Eliot, *The Waste Land*).

My friend's book presented a new opportunity, I reasoned with myself. This was fiction—not criticism—so I should be able to grasp it more easily. I wanted so much to celebrate his achievement, but after weeks of trying to read his book, always stymied by the first few pages, I finally gave up. Only much later would I realize that it wasn't the pain alone, but rather all of the medications I was taking that made it so impossible to read, lulling me into a cocooned, cloudy haze, a cotton-balled insulation that dulled the pain somewhat but made it impossible for me to think coherently.

I also felt lost without my work identity. In London, even with the onset of my headaches, I had made major strides in what I had hoped would be my "big book." Motivated and inspired, I ambitiously imagined that this book would secure for me the title of full professor. I was looking forward to another twenty, even twenty-five, good years of teaching and writing, savoring the notion that, unlike nearly every other profession, that of academe actually allows one to get better with age— professors' pedagogical skills in the classroom become more fine-tuned, their mentoring of students becomes more creative, and their own writing takes on layers of density and connection possible only after years of writing and research.

I now feared that my old career would never again be the same. It wasn't ambition so much as longing that drove these worries. My friend Kris wisely counseled, "Hope for the best, but prepare for the worst." I would have to hope to get back as much of my ability in the classroom—the energy, doggedness, and intensity—as necessary to inspire ninety New York City students each semester to love poetry (or at least not to loathe it—and me). I would also have to hope to have the stamina to finish the two languishing manuscripts that littered my library and on which I had expended hours of effort already. I also began preparing myself for the possibility that I would never be able to write scholarly criticism again. In the first six months of pain, I didn't even walk into my library—what was the point? The unread books (necessary reads to stay abreast in my field), the nearly finished manuscript on John Milton's poetry, the fully researched and unwritten articles that a year earlier had seemed so timely, so relevant, and the thousands of documents representing three years of research that I had gathered for my big book all lay untouched. Was it time to admit to myself that perhaps that work would remain unfinished?

The worst moment for me, the one I considered the nadir of my professional career, occurred later that year when I had to back out nearly at the last minute from an academic conference in London to which I had been invited. For me, being invited, rather than sending in a paper to be accepted, felt like a new stage of recognition in my field. As my friend Amanda summed up the situation in one of her pithy adages, "You were invited to the party, and you want to go to the party, but right now, sweetie, you just can't go to the party."

CHAPTER 10

Mind and Body

It was also my violent heart that broke,
falling down the front hall stairs. . . .
The fracture was twice. The fracture was double.
The days are horizontal. The days are a drag.
—ANNE SEXTON, *from* "The Break"

Sexton's autobiographical poem describes a period of incapacitation after having broken her hip; what intrigues me most about the poem is how she makes explicit the connection between the mind and body. A mental breakdown accompanied her physical breakdown; and the lines of the poem mirror this double break, as they fracture into two sentences. What I also find interesting is how she describes her mental agitation and physical pain as occurring simultaneously, rather than one break leading to the other. I was not so sure that this chronology was the case for me.

Doctors had begun to question me on this chronology as well, suggesting that my mental perturbation was causing my physical problems, rather than the other way around. The causes of chronic daily headaches are multitudinous and, in individual cases, notoriously difficult to identify. The main causes are neuropathic pain (damage to either a peripheral nerve or the central nervous system), nociceptive injuries to the body's soft tissue, psychogenic pain (some form of psychological distress), or often a combination of these factors.

Because tension and depression do not simply exacerbate but, in some cases, actually cause chronic daily headaches, eventually some doctors gently (and others more aggressively) began to probe at appointments, "Were you unhappy in London? Anxious? Have you experienced greater tension or depression in recent months?" After these appointments, I would think, so these doctors believe that these headaches are not just literally in my head but also because of my head? If one shrank my head, would my pain also shrink?

At first, I was defensive, even indignant; but, insidiously, once doctors raised the issue, I began to wonder if they were correct. It became a classic chicken-or-the-egg preoccupation. Which had come first—physical pain leading to mental pain—or vice versa? Perhaps underlying dissatisfactions, long-stifled grief, or stress accounted for this pain? The summer in London had been difficult—the work arduous and lonely. Is that why I had cracked? If one's life felt fragmented, could one so internalize fragmentation so as to break oneself? Certainly, the longer this surreal existence continued, the more stressed out and depressed I felt. No Cartesian split separated my body and mind at present; my physical and psychological pain seemed interchangeable.

These questions tortured me. My mind a labyrinth, I got tangled. My thoughts a-mazed. I knew why, of course. Just lying there, my brain had nothing else to do but fixate on my pain. In this way, the mind and body of a person in pain are not connected at all but radically disconnected, as the desires and agency of the mind conflict fundamentally with the inability of the body. The mind tortures itself, and this ongoing emotional melodrama cannot reconcile itself to the physical stasis engendered by the pain. The rapid shifts and cascades of emotional responses to the pain are turbulent: while the body remains inert, the mind is swept into one tidal wave after the next. On some days, nothing else occupies my mind but the all-consuming pain. I find that the energy required to gird myself mentally through a pain spike leaves me utterly depleted to handle anything else. Other days, I find myself obsessing about how all I do is obsess about my pain, thereby creating for myself new difficulties, problems, and self-defeating doubts.

This tendency, I think, is one of the hardest things for people who don't have chronic pain to understand. Merely spectators, they reason, "You have to change your attitude. You need a better mental outlook to overcome this pain." Of course what they fail to understand is that the sufferer has already been thinking the same thing—blaming and punishing himself for not having found it possible to overcome the pain or, worse, to do anything else but overcome the pain. Nevertheless, I kept instinctively rejecting the too pat conclusion that psychological pain had somehow led to my physical pain. Before the summer in London, I had felt pretty darn good.

In December, I went to a new pain anesthesiologist. Humane and kind, he listened to my narrative quietly, patiently. When I finished speaking, he paused and then dramatically announced that my pain was "classic C2 pain." The pain that started in my neck and shot through my head corresponded to the pathway of the C2 nerve. He pulled out a plastic model of the cervical spine and showed me how the nerve jutted out along each side of the vertebra at its periphery. Rubbery, like a worm, the nerve looked so vulnerable, so easily prone to damage by an unstable bone. Nerve pain is referred; it moves. The pathway of C2 pain is directly through the center of the head. I remember feeling elated—finally, finally, there was a definitive name for my pain and even a cure, as he informed me that he did in fact have the expertise, unlike the first doctor, to burn this nerve. This diagnosis had an immediate, if short-lived, effect on my emotional state. It brought my self-flagellation temporarily to an end as this new doctor eased my doubts, confirming that my physical pain had caused my mental anguish and not the other way around.

The new doctor would first perform a temporary diagnostic block on both the left and right side of the C2 nerve. If I had a significant reduction in pain, then he would perform the more long-lasting bilateral medial branch nerve rhizotomy using pulsed radiofrequency thermocoagulation (or RF ablation). This procedure differed from the burning technique used by the first doctor, as it would not damage the nerve itself (one of the risks, I learned, of the by now, apparently, antiquated phenol block). The RF ablation would set up an electromagnetic field that would eventually stun the nerve's signaling devices to the brain. The benefits of the procedure could generally last for as long as four to six months. It would take four to six weeks for the electromagnetic field to work efficiently; nevertheless, I calculated, that would mean approximately two and a half months out of four or four and a half months out of six to be free from these headaches. One could continually repeat the procedure, and sometimes a series of these procedures could permanently break the pain cycle.

For my family this felt like the watershed moment. My mother and Eric accompanied me to the first merely diagnostic procedure. The doctor gave me antianxiety medication before the procedure and did the shots on both sides in the same day. For a man who wields needles for a living, he has one of the gentlest touches I've ever known in a doctor. At one point when I whispered, "I hate this," he softly responded, "I know you do. And you're doing great." His empathic bedside manner alone proved him to be the best doctor I had met thus far, and his skills and procedures were light-years ahead of my first doctor's. The definitiveness of both the diagnosis and his technique led to an equally definitive improvement in my mood. Filled again with hope, I breezed through the procedure.

Afterward, my mother whisked me back to her apartment, gently placing an ice pack on my neck. Excited, she quizzed me for hours after: "How is the pain level now?" "What about now?" "Any better?" And, indeed, my pain levels did seem to go down for four hours. The new pain doctor, in light of these results, recommended a bilateral RF ablation of my C2 nerves. The breakthrough had finally arrived! I would be cured.

CHAPTER 11

Advice

The [patients'] eyes are fixed to me. But no darkness
would recover them, no alley make them male again—
Don't look at me, I am not fiction—
They were men once
but there is no proof of it now.
Unreal now, they brood over old skirmishes.

Like them I am drifting into fiction.
Like them I will be injected with heat and ice.
This morning, sweating, I await my fate
typed out onto a green form.
What further fiction is being imagined. What fee?
　　—JOYCE CAROL OATES, from "How I Became Fiction"

Days before I was to have the RF ablation procedure, Eric spoke with an eminent neurosurgeon who, unfortunately, did not live in New York. He had some initial observations about my situation but advised us to visit him for a proper consultation. Eric and I decided temporarily to postpone the RF ablation, as the doctor and his team could see me the following week.

I met with the neurosurgeon, the "quarterback" of my case, only after a full day of tests—more blood work, more X-rays, more examinations. One particularly ingenious X-ray was taken by placing the camera directly into my open mouth. The technician showed me on the film how he had gotten a perfect view of the fractured dens from this angle. I then had individual consultations with a neurologist who specialized in head pain, a pain management doctor, and a psychopharmacologist.

The day ended in a long consultation with the neurosurgeon, who by now had gathered my background information and test results. All of my scans hung outside the door of the examining room in long rows. Peeking through a crack in the door, we watched fascinated as a team of doctors pored over these scans for half an hour, before we finally met the neurosurgeon.

I was "drifting into fiction," surely, as he spun yet another tale to explain my condition. In his estimable opinion, the unfused C2 fracture did indeed account for my pain. Because the bone was unstable, it was constantly bombarding the nerve. Further, the three millimeters of instability were dangerous. While I had been lucky that nothing catastrophic had occurred in the last twenty-two years, there was no guarantee that in a future accident I would be so lucky. He did not find my "soft story" so unusual. While my body had functioned for years with a skeletal, or "mechanical," defect, my body could no longer withstand it. He finally thought that after all of the anti-inflammatories, physical therapy, and injections that I had already tried, I had exhausted all reasonable efforts to stabilize the pain.

He then advised the most radical fiction yet to effect a recovery. From both a structural and pain perspective, he recommended C1-C2 fusion surgery to stabilize the bone. The surgeon could take bone from my hip, graft it onto the vertebrae, and then hold it in place with both screws and wiring. Eventually, the two separate vertebrae would fuse together into one bone. The instability would be eliminated and, hopefully, the pain too, as the bone would no longer bang into and exacerbate nerves and other soft tissue.

I had heard that the doctor was quite conservative and usually turned away prospective surgical candidates. Even if he deemed the surgery necessary, he would often refer the patient to another doctor who could competently handle it. So when he suggested that he would be willing to perform the surgery himself, I interpreted his opinion not only as definitive but also as indicative of the delicacy of my situation. I supposed that he must have thought that his skills and level of expertise were needed to perform this surgery. I agreed on the spot to have him conduct the surgery, even though his first available surgery date was not for another two and a half months.

I returned to New York and had time to make only one further appointment, a consultation with my new pain anesthesiologist. Had he ever, I asked, seen a nerve after spinal fusion surgery remain exacerbated? He said no but insisted that his practice consisted of patients already deemed nonsurgical candidates. He offered to arrange for one of the neurosurgeons affiliated with his hospital to provide a more definitive second opinion on the question of fusion surgery.

This not second but rather fourth, even fifth, opinion would not take place. An unexpected cancellation in the neurosurgeon's schedule opened up an imminent surgery date for me, if I wanted it—December 19, only a few days away. This date could not have been more propitious, coinciding beautifully with our children's winter vacation. Their academic work and daily routines would therefore not suffer without their parents around. The pieces further fell into place as Eric's parents offered to take Benjamin and Lilly to Florida. A windfall for the children; they would get a real vacation in the sun surrounded by the extended family. Even our dog, Charlie, would be taken care of, as our babysitter Cora agreed to watch him. As we rushed forward, we never once doubted my decision to have the surgery or my speed in making this decision.

CHAPTER 12

Surgery

Rose is a rose is a rose is a rose.
—GERTRUDE STEIN, from "Sacred Emily"

Surgery is surgery is surgery is surgery. That is, the word itself lays bare its associations, its attendant emotions and connotations. It is what it is. Risk. Difficulty. Vulnerability. Attendant Pain. A Body Altered. The only relevant question is whether the surgery heals or merely disfigures the body.

The first encounter I had at the hospital concerned payment for the surgery—seventy-five thousand dollars to be exact. A financial transaction, after all, this service demanded remuneration. I dutifully proffered my precertification numbers and insurance identification cards, more concerned for all the thousands of people without medical insurance in this country than for myself at this point. The attendant then asked whether I had a living will and, if so, whether I had brought my copy. This had not occurred to me before I left New York, and the question unsettled me. I got a bit teary, and my sister kept her arm around me while I filled out the paperwork: no artificial or heroic efforts to keep this shell of a body alive, if there was no reasonable expectation of my recovery. Yes, please do give away any and all of my organs, if they could be of use to others. My family thought I was being morbid; I thought that I was merely responding to the hospital's protocol. A psychologist then prepped me for the surgery, warning that this surgery was difficult—indeed, the "most painful" surgery one can have—and then reminded me, again, of the risks. "Yes, yes, I know—death, paralysis, et cetera, et cetera, I get it," I responded. In greater detail, the doctor also described how this procedure would necessarily diminish, quite substantially, movement of my neck, both from side to side and up and down. Another bit of forewarning that my mind managed to evade—flitting into a nether region in which it would not have to take such a consequence into account.

I only received one other bit of unexpected news. The doctor would have to shave off some of my hair for the surgery. For some reason, I became fixated on this. Why the permanent consequence of radically reduced movement in my neck made no impression and the temporary consequence of cut hair so upset me, I have no logical explanation. My mind, at any rate, now had something on which to obsess: Where was the surgeon going to slice? Why did he need access to where my hair grew? Where indeed was this fusion to take place? I thought it was just going to be in my neck. The resident explained that the slice would begin at my neck and end at the level of my ears, about four inches in length. I hadn't fully understood the physiology until that moment and became alarmed. My only recourse for my belated second thoughts was a piece of paper taped to my chest as I was being wheeled into surgery. Scrawled by my sister Jeanne at the last minute, it read: "Please do not shave off more hair than you have to."

In the time leading up to surgery, this predicament at least engendered some comic relief. We had an enormous laugh, wondering why we had worried so much about the doctor's surgical experience when we really should have been wondering about how good a haircut he gave. I said that I would have traded the entire family being with me at the hospital for my haircutter. Why hadn't he come with me to the hospital?

I was still smiling when the attendant wheeled me away, but the atmosphere soon chilled all humor. Left alone against the wall of the operating room with only a thin sheet covering me, I shivered. How many times in these months had I faced the cold blast of hospitals? Giant freezers, the hospitals preserved me in a state akin to frozen food. I had been stocked away, my life iced,

while I waited for the defrosting to thaw me. Feeling dehuman-
ized, the frozen spinach next to the more interesting T-bones, I
waited, completely ignored, as a dozen people whizzed around
me preparing the operating room. I had only a brief instant of
feeling like the main course, when they finally wheeled me to the
center of the room; but they wanted a carcass, not a thinking
being, and quickly added anesthesia to my IV.

Five hours later, I woke up and once again had the semblance
of agency. A nurse gave me a "patient-controlled intravenous
analgesia," that is, a computerized pump that allowed me to push
a button to receive morphine. The nurse warned, "Patients like
to monitor their own pain, but no one else is allowed to push the
button for you. You can't overdose yourself, as only a certain
prescribed amount will be administered." At first, remembering
how morphine made me throw up all those years ago, I said that
I didn't want it. Once I was reassured that they would administer
a medication to counteract nausea at the same time, I gladly
clutched at the pump.

Apparently I hold the record in that wing of the hospital for
clicking the pump so many times in one night—392 times, to be
exact. An Addict Is Born.

Jeanne, it seems, had trouble watching me in the early days
after surgery. She kept leaning over and clicking the button herself. Jeanne, stubborn, and Eric, ever the rule player, got into
several tiffs over this tendency. Jeanne and my mother also did a
fair amount of yelling at the doctors and nurses, I think because
they found it so unbearable to watch me in so much pain. I only
screamed at one resident, who roughly woke me up out of a dead
sleep at 5:00 a.m. two days after the surgery without even the
decency of a "good morning." The neurosurgeon, miffed at my
rudeness, later suggested that I ought to appreciate how hard
everyone worked at the hospital and try to check my misbehavior
in the future. He also implied that I should apologize to the
resident, rather than the other way around. As our friend Kris
e-mailed to Eric, "That hospital has no idea what has hit them.

Those Greenbergs are formidable." We were a handful for the staff.

I didn't care a rat's ass.

I was miserable, a grotesque and leaking body. Too shocked by the pain levels even to cry, to talk, to complain, I lay for the first day with eyes closed, whimpering, not moving, except to click the morphine pump. My sister Jackie wanted to help me clean my teeth with a wet swab. Honestly, my teeth were the least of my worries. Instead, she inserted ice chips sideways into my mouth, which I found difficult to open. My tongue, rank with horror, remained mute.

On the second day of my "recovery," I opened my eyes for the first time but couldn't focus. Seeing only blurred shapes, light, and shadows, I had to close my eyes again. At first, I was so out of it, I didn't even realize that I had a problem. When this pattern kept recurring, on the third day, I finally said to one of the doctors, "I don't think that I can see." Within minutes, the room became busy with more doctors, lengthy questioning, and eye tests.

It seems that I had effectively gone blind. Whether this was a permanent condition, an unanticipated consequence of the surgery, or a temporary one, my neurosurgeon seemed unwilling to discuss. This was the only time in the entire year that Eric lost it. Unbeknownst to me at the time, he blamed himself for allowing me to rush into surgery and was beside himself with worry. I too worried but, oddly, felt more resignation than any other emotion. I thought, Of course, the car accident has obliterated a second sense—first smell and now sight. Having felt oddly victimized for so many months, I submitted to yet another sensory loss, another physical deprivation. I found it perversely comforting that I was not alone. Look at Milton, I thought, and, isn't it at least a little coincidental that Persephone's name roughly means "the absence of light"?

After another twenty-four hours of blindness, the doctor insisted that I visit the hospital's eye clinic for a thorough examination. The eye clinic must have been a mile away from my hospital room, and even though my neck and chin were encased since the surgery in a hard plastic brace, I cringed and gasped at every bump we encountered. With my catheter bag in plain view and the IV pole dragging behind me, I half sat, half drooped, in the wheelchair, dressed only in a flimsy hospital gown. I had never felt so freaky.

It was at this point that the story became truly farcical. Eric received a call from Cora while we were speeding through the miles of enclosed tunnels toward the eye clinic. She was sobbing on the phone. Eric couldn't even understand at first what she was saying but soon learned that our dog Charlie had out of nowhere gotten sick after our departure. Cora had taken him to the vet only to discover that he had advanced liver cancer and was dying. The vet had counseled that neither surgery nor chemotherapy could save him. She had only two choices—either put him to sleep immediately, since he was suffering, or inject him with steroid shots to keep him alive long enough for our family to say good-bye to him in person.

Poor, shocked Eric. I tried to lighten the situation, joking with him that, if he knew what was good for him, he would immediately put us both out of our misery. He looked wretched but tried to humor me. He countered that he would opt for injections to keep Charlie alive but that, if I continued to be so annoying, he might have to take me up on my suggestion. For the time being, though, he kept marching me toward the eye clinic.

Recovery

I wasn't permanently blind, the eye doctor pronounced. Apparently my eyes were heading in opposite directions, and the doctor had managed to trick them briefly into alignment again. She said that I had only temporarily lost the ability to focus and attributed this condition to the amount of morphine I was self-administering. She cautioned that I would remain unfocused until I stopped the drug. In response, the doctors drastically reduced the amount of morphine I was permitted, but for the next three days in the hospital, I refused to give up the clicker, "blindness regained," as long as it meant that I felt less pain.

On day seven of my recovery, my now stern neurosurgeon ordered me to give up the pump. When I tried wheedling and cajoling, "Just two more hits today, really, just two more," his patience ran out. He admitted that I'd had a rough recovery, but he insisted that, as I was checking out of the hospital the next day, I needed to transition to oral medications. No more morphine—Just Say No. So I relinquished the pump, blindness lost and pain regained, and sent Eric immediately out to the pharmacy to fill all of my new prescriptions: Valium to relax the muscles in my neck and a panoply of opioid pain medications, including Dilaudid and Percocet. I was supposed to wind down these painkillers over the course of the next few weeks and stay on Valium for at least ten weeks to avoid muscle spasms in my neck.

As I began regaining strength, though, our dog began slipping further. Cora called again to say that the injection had not revived him but rather had made him worse. Suffering, he was now too sick to move, unable to walk, stand, or eat. Panged, Eric and I thought it was cruel to keep him alive until we returned, and Eric arranged to have him put to sleep that same day.

The dog's death was interpreted differently by each member of our family. Our Peruvian babysitter saw his death as an act of God. She described how, in many South American countries, traditional beliefs still maintain that a sacrifice of one life is needed in order to preserve another life; therefore, Charlie had to die in order for my life to be spared. I, ironically, felt heartbroken over a pet who had routinely engendered asthma attacks during his lifetime and began making plans to acquire another dog as soon as possible. For my sister Jeanne, also allergic to the dog, his death was a relief. She reasoned that not having asthma problems would make my recovery easier. Eric and I knew that for our children Charlie's death would be traumatic.

Sitting in the hospital cafeteria "enjoying" our Christmas leftovers—the usual assortment of overcooked vegetables, desiccated chicken and Jell-O—amid patients and families equally miserable, we began arranging what to do about Benjamin and Lilly. We finally decided that, even though I was somewhat precarious, we should fly down to Florida to tell them about Charlie in person. A phone call just didn't seem adequate: "Happy New Year, kids. Your dog is dead."

We left for Florida a few days later. Traveling was difficult, but arriving in Boca Raton, Florida, on New Year's Eve, with the children so thrilled, made the trip wholly worth it. This reunion was so lovely that we didn't have the heart to tell them about Charlie until the next day.

As we had expected, Benjamin and Lilly took the loss hard. How to console two innocents, torn between weeping for their pet and dousing themselves in the blissful chill of the pool? A day of mourning felt absurd in the tropical heat. What we had not anticipated was how this loss would become a touchstone for Lilly. Even now, she remains fixated on Charlie's death and still occasionally breaks into sobs at the mere mention of his name. She has come to refer to this period a.p. (after pain) as "the worst time in her life." When asked why, she itemizes two reasons: first, because her dog died, and, second, because of her mom's neck. My (perhaps erroneous) theory for why the dog takes priority is that he has become a potent metaphor, as if she has transplanted all of the trauma and emotional upheaval of the year onto the loss of her beloved Charlie. Somehow, I imagine, she has subconsciously analogized the grief of having lost her former mother to the grief of having lost her dog. How else for a little girl to process the unwanted changes in her life, her worries about the health of those she loves, and the real losses she has had to face? Perhaps it has been easier for her to latch on to this tangible loss rather than the more amorphous and, in this period, unspoken loss of a mommy.

Again, the myth of Persephone, so much about the mourning mothers and daughters must face in the wake of each other's absences, resonates with such clarity in my life. How to miss someone with whom one shares the deepest of human bonds when that person is technically not gone? Like Persephone, I was only half there; but perhaps, when Lilly had come to expect the whole of me, having only a part made the loss all the more frustrating for her.

Boca Raton otherwise proved uneventful and predictable—weather ever sunny; the slightly mildewing, cheesy condominium unchanged in the past twenty years; the strip malls lining the highway perpetually bland. The only difference is that I had changed. Suddenly, I fit right into the retirement community where Eric's parents had their condominium. My lung age, according to my asthma doctor, was that of a sixty-four-year-old woman. My bone density, according to my radiologist, was that of a sixty-five-year-old woman. And, now, my neck brace announced that I too had had fusion surgery.

Apparently, everyone's cervical spine had deteriorated in Boca, as one senior citizen after the next came up to me throughout the week—at meals, by the pool, in the shopping center—eager to discuss the gory details of their own fusion surgeries and to commiserate with me about the difficulty of the recovery. One woman actually lifted up her hair to show me how she was wearing a fake hair extension to cover where the doctor had shaved off her hair. She enthusiastically wrote down the name of the store where she had purchased this extension and advised me to get one, too. "The hair is fake," she gushed, as if this were a bonus, "so they can dye the hair to match your own hair color." Her scar looked like she had been through a shredder, and her doctor had shaved off nearly all the bottom half of her hair. I felt newly beholden to the expertise of my neurosurgeon. You could barely see where he had made his incisions or shaved my hair, apparently a better hairdresser than we had thought. One bit of advice from a retiree did prove helpful. One man swore by a special orthopedic pillow that could be purchased at the neighboring mall (on Butts Road, I kid not) in a store that sold only items for the cervical spine. That pillow has proven invaluable, and I don't go anywhere without it.

CHAPTER 14

Loneliness

I'm Nobody! Who are you?
Are you—Nobody—Too?
Then there's a pair of us?
Don't tell! they'd advertise—you know!

How dreary—to be—Somebody!
How public—like a Frog—
To tell one's name—the livelong June—
To an admiring Bog!
    —EMILY DICKINSON, No. 288

⌐⁓⁓ I have read several "survival" memoirs written by famous individuals, Somebodies, in Dickinson's parlance, who underwent a terrible trauma and recovered, even if only partially. What I find striking about these memoirs is how unselfconsciously they name-drop and offhandedly mention being beset by visitors (usually famous ones), prayed for in congregations nationwide, and overwhelmed by the many cards, flowers, even casseroles received not only from friends and colleagues but also from complete strangers. This connectedness to the outside world must have provided them with a sense of community and reconfirmed their public and professional identities.

This was not the case for me; reclusive, most comfortable with a few close, intimate friendships rather than with the larger world of acquaintances, living the necessarily solitary life of an academic—I clearly am a Nobody. Further, pain is by its nature isolating. The mind already finds itself trapped, incarcerated in the carcass of a once-functional body, and doubly isolated, as no one healthy can understand what it is like to live in constant pain. The psychological and emotional contours of this state create a kind of existential solitude.

On the most basic level, so many of my days in the classroom had been filled with conversation, and I found myself missing the unique collaboration that occurs between teachers and students. Adrienne Rich describes loneliness in a particularly rich image that both replicates what I now found myself missing in my life and illustrates why. She writes in "Song":

> *If I'm lonely*
> *it's with the rowboat ice-fast on the shore*
> *in the last red light of the year*
> *that knows what it is, that knows it's neither*
> *ice nor mud nor winter light*
> *but wood, with a gift for burning*

A reader quickly grasps the way in which feeling alone, isolated, superfluous, has something in common with a rowboat stuck out of the water. In the classroom, this image has the capacity to expand as more minds begin teasing out its meanings. One student riffs on why the light is red—the color of fire, perhaps. Another student points out that the wood boat is like the lonely heart. Excited by this analogy, students begin associating the fire with passion, heat, erotic love. Then, the class itself gets heated, and students start disagreeing with one another. One student observes that the boat is vulnerable to fire, while another student insists that without such fire, the heart/boat is frozen, unable to fulfill its purpose, even dead. By allowing the metaphor to breathe in this way, not only the boat but also our own hearts thaw; we relate to the poem's speaker and thereby feel less lonely ourselves. In this period of my life, without such classroom conversations, I now found myself cold, lifeless, useless—lonely.

I also found myself freezing for warmth, camaraderie, burning friendships; but my body, let alone my mind, made such intimacy difficult. My relationship with my husband most profoundly changed, our roles radically altering as the months progressed. Gone were the familiar roles of husband and friend, as he became nurse, parent figure, angel of mercy. How as a couple, or as individuals, we fared during these months of forced separation remained unspoken. We avoided the topic—he, out of natural reticence and probably a desire not to hurt or distress me further, and I, out of embarrassment, lonely for contact but also wholly unable to handle it.

As the months progressed, my social world also shrank. So many acquaintances, work colleagues, and fellow parents at our children's school seemed to vanish. Or, had I, as in Dickinson's poem, been "banish[ed]"? On the infrequent occasions when I emerged from my hermit's existence, acquaintances initially asked the usual questions: "How are you?" I would answer, "The same." "Any improvement?" "No." Then I would feel the silent judgment: what a bore she is. And, at the next near meeting, I would greet, instead of questions, a ducked head as the person scurried away from me. I was a leper or, perhaps, merely the accountant—predictable, vaguely distasteful, joyless. Who wouldn't avoid me?

I did receive a few e-mails, calls, and flowers from unexpected acquaintances, and these rare events would so tap into my insecurity that I found myself inordinately prizing them. Rereading and printing even the smallest of such e-mails, I clutched them in an effort to temper my growing sense of isolation and loneliness. A few friendships didn't survive. One friend with whom I had been close for more than twenty years called but only after insistent prodding from my mother. She has not called since, and I nurse that wound that has no stitches or bandages to assuage it.

Petulant whining aside, I am acutely aware that, while I might not have had the most popular year in my life, I, nevertheless, received an outpouring of love and support from both steadfast family members and friends. My two sisters, Jeanne and Jackie, took to visiting me each and every weekend, no matter how busy they were. They would arrive with some helpful bit of information—the name of a good personal trainer or a healing center—anecdotes from the outside world to amuse me;

a beautiful blouse to hide the swelling from the surgery; or an hour session with a reflexologist. They came over to provide me with moral support and also to help with Lilly and Benjamin. Countless times throughout the year they would take the kids on special outings, help them with their homework, or buy them the necessaries I had been unable to purchase.

My lifelong friends were also loyal to a fault: calling regularly, e-mailing, checking in, and traveling sometimes long distances in order to visit me. Audrey and Tamir traveled from Westchester regularly, simply to sit in chairs next to my bed and let me cry. My friend Jillisa visited from Chicago, selfless enough to be content with seeing only the interior of my house and never even making it into Manhattan during her trip. To my Manhattan friends, coming to Brooklyn had always been psychologically rather than physically daunting. (We were only one subway stop away from Manhattan after all, I often teased them.) Those friends who had never made it to our home now made the trek on a regular basis (complaining bitterly, of course, but only in order to generate a laugh). They would bring food, and we would have a dinner party in my bed.

I derived my daily strength, support, and guffaws from Lisa, Amanda, Susan, and Leslie, the "coffee girls," so named because, after school drop-offs in the morning for the last ten years, we have regularly met at Starbucks for coffee and chatter. They willingly allowed the venue to shift to my bedroom in the early days a.p., so that I could avoid the walk to Starbucks. In my room, they would flop onto the bed with me, open the shades so that I could no longer remain buried in the dark, freely go into my closet trying on loot, and generally yank me out of my cave. They installed themselves in my house on those mornings and emotionally have never left me. Nevertheless, when the bewitching hour, 10:00 a.m., came, my friends would disperse to attend to their busy lives, and I would wonder what to do for the rest of the day.

My family, luckily, seemed to be faring better than I on this front, their lives remaining busy and social. Eric's job is relent-lessly filled with people. He receives on average sixty phone calls and at least one hundred e-mails a day. It's hard to feel lonely with that amount of human interaction. In this period of crisis, his ABC colleagues, like an enormous family, all rallied even more tightly around him, lavishly spoiling us with meals, flowers, cards, notes, thoughtful presents, offers of help, and constant e-mail check-ins to see how we were coping. I must have dictated nearly eighty thank-you notes to his colleagues, many of whom I had never met, in the first six months of my injury alone.

Benjamin too remained his usual effervescent self. He would pounce on my bed in the weeks after surgery, give me a brief back rub, and, with an exaggerated groan, roll over and announce, "My turn!" He was extremely affectionate with me and, like his father, showed unflinching optimism about my future prog-nosis. He constantly told me that he loved me, was proud of my bravery, and reassured me that I would definitely, definitely get better!

Mostly, though, I noticed that he had somehow managed to remove himself from the emotional Sturm und Drang of our household. Typical, I think, of most seventh graders, his life began to revolve around his gang of friends that year. He spent as much time with them as possible, often outside, practicing skateboarding or playing football and arriving home every Fri-day afternoon with them to eat pizza and play video games.

He also managed to distance himself further from me, find-ing his identity and spirit galvanized by interactions not only with his friends but also with his father and extended family of male relatives who organized special activities and trips for him. My father took him skiing. They braved black diamonds all day and played gin rummy, backgammon, and chess every evening. His uncle Jonny took Benjamin on weekly golf excursions, re-plete with stops in Coney Island to get Nathan's hot dogs, which they emphatically insisted were the best in New York. Captain Nick, as he is affectionately called, another uncle, made regular fishing and boating dates with Benjamin throughout the year and also took him skiing, and Uncle David palled around with Benjamin the entire Christmas vacation, letting Benjamin join his all-adult, eighteen-hole golf games.

Sweet Lilly, like Benjamin, also began turning outward and became more independent. She showed reserves of inner strength and courage that astounded not only me but even her teachers. Her midyear report card spoke more about their respect for and admiration of her character than of her academic work. I was particularly touched by their references to her compassion. Instead of clinging to me, as she always had in the past, my shy mama's girl, she began to form deeper and deeper relationships with her friends, teachers, and other members of the family. Lilly had always refused to go on playdates at other children's houses, and we had become used to having our house filled with girls on any given day, but I had to change the rules in the fall. Bad shot days led me to put our house into temporary quarantine; I didn't want her friends to see me like that. On bad pain days, I also found myself severely phonosensitive. The giggling, shrieking, and happy feet prancing up and down the stairs were too much for me. On those days, Lilly had of necessity to go to other people's houses if she was going to have a playdate. This move into independence I welcomed, feeling particularly happy when I heard how she had bonded not only with the girls but also with their mothers. I felt comforted, as I am sure Lilly did, knowing that she had mommy substitutes on whom to lean.

As my family remained intact and absorbed in their external lives, I felt both relief—and a worse form of loneliness. They had all found other attachments, while I remained isolated in bed, wondering how to fill the fourteen empty hours that yawned before me every waking day.

CHAPTER 15

Retail Therapy

. . . fevers of shopping
—a kind of excitement for her
but also a bandage
over bewilderment
*   —*ADRIENNE RICH, from "Plaza Street and Flatbush"

    All of the women in my family are beautiful, with high cheekbones, gaminelike features, and lissome frames; and while I share a certain number of these attributes, no one has ever considered me one of the beauties of my family. That rarefied prize belongs to my grandmother Lillian, mother, two lovely sisters, cousins Lilly and Kricky, and daughter Lilly—Graces each and every one of them.

Looking in the mirror after surgery, I was depressed to see that I had moved even farther from this ideal. The surgeon had required that I wear a neck brace for ten weeks postsurgery. The white plastic brace locked my neck into an immovable position; I couldn't do the simplest things, walk down the stairs by myself, or tie my shoelaces. The neck brace, so unsightly and ungainly, I couldn't hide even under Eric's largest turtleneck sweater.

My chin and cheeks flabbily overflowed the edge of the brace, and I appeared to have no cheekbones at all. My skin also seemed to have lost all of its elasticity, gathering in elephantine folds that, in turn, caused the edges of my mouth to droop. I looked like I was perpetually frowning. Friends my own age were beginning to develop laugh lines, a crinkling at the sides of their eyes and mouths that proclaimed a life well spent in gaiety. I worried that my gathering wrinkles instead bespoke misery. To hell with paradise lost. I was now experiencing youth lost, beauty lost.

And dignity lost. Women in our family adhere to rigorous grooming habits and pride ourselves on our eccentric clothing and personal style. It functions as a particularly trustworthy and long-accepted form of armor to gird ourselves against the world. No matter how bad one might feel, it was not acceptable also to look bad. Yet, here I was, frizzy, messy, bloody, wrinkly. I couldn't even get a haircut (how would I lean back in the chair?) and so had taken to cutting my own bangs. They used to curve gently upward at the edges, a cheerful smiley face above my eyes. My own shearing led instead to the bangs sloping dramatically downward and ending in a point like an eagle's beak at the center of my forehead. Taking a shower was a major ordeal, altogether not worth the effort, as shampoo trickled into and burned the incision on my neck. Worse even than dirty, I was puffy and black and blue all over. The swelling from my hip was so extreme I couldn't wear my normal clothes. For weeks, of necessity, I wore net, disposable underpants provided by the hospital and, in addition to Eric's sweaters, loose sweatpants with elasticized waistbands. Less a Grace, I more resembled an old hag.

The surgeon at this time strongly urged me to get out of bed and start walking every day to keep up my strength, but, bedridden, I hadn't walked in months. To my brittle, shaky legs, walking was a formidable effort. It also proved excessively painful—tiptoeing, gliding, and shuffling were the only ways of perambulating without sending pain waves into my head. Further, it was a typical New York winter replete with bone-chilling winds and icy sidewalks. How and where was I supposed to walk?

With a preternatural instinct, I figured it out—enclosed malls. Reminded of the many Saturdays spent mall hopping during my teens, I found myself able to hobble for hours in these enclosed walkways. I became creative at finding ever-new ones just on the outskirts of the city. My sister, who also grew up mall roaming, has a philosophy, if you will, about malls. You walk with a partner, chatting incessantly, and only stop for the occasional sweet treat (at a conveniently located Godiva shop) or cosmetics (a little female pampering), but one must never, ever linger in stores, let alone try on clothing. The pleasure is in the pure amble.

I am afraid that here I went terribly awry. Ambling, I did not. Shopping, I did—in earnest. I took to spending extravagant amounts of money that we simply didn't have on designer clothing that I had no reason to wear. My days so without meaning or purpose led me to create little inventions of lives. I could pretend that I had a career that demanded the perfect Prada suit and a social life that required the beautiful Chloé cocktail dress. Months later, I am embarrassed to admit, I still had not gone back to work or out to a party, and most of these newly purchased outfits still hung in my closet unworn.

The only person to whom I would even confess to these shopping frenzies was a friend who works at a fashion magazine. A true expert in the field of fashion, she could discuss with authority the merits of my purchases. We would heatedly debate whether a dress would look too young, too short, or too faddish on me and whether a particular Lanvin necklace had already proven a classic (honestly, I finally have enough clear-sightedness now to admit the absurdity of purchasing an expensive necklace when my entire neck and chest were encased in plastic).

She called my purchases retail therapy, and in the empty days after surgery, these purchases did fill a particular need. They shored me up and kept nihilistic thoughts at bay. I could distract myself with pretty objects, simply by ogling the delicate filigree of the jewelry and the silky fabrics of the designer clothing.

My purchases too stemmed from my feelings of deprivation. With so few pleasures open to me, I found myself seduced by the American consumer dream. Lulled by the piped-in music, the crowds of happy post-Christmas shoppers, the January sale prices, the perfectly heated artificial terrain, I felt more relaxed, serene even. While Adrienne Rich's imagined woman found shopping a "bandage over bewilderment," my shopping had become so excessive that I was creating a veritable pharmacy of psychologically buoying "medical" supplies. Shopping offered me crutches over crying, wheelchairs over overwhelm, braces bracing me. Although I still felt every step ricochet into my head, the shopping temporarily allayed my worries and loneliness and staved off feelings of living in a wasteland.

CHAPTER 16

Things Fall Apart

Turning and turning in the widening gyre
The falcon cannot hear the falconer;
Things fall apart; the centre cannot hold. . . .
Surely the Second Coming is at hand. . . .
And what rough beast, its hour come round at last,
Slouches towards Bethlehem to be born?
—WILLIAM BUTLER YEATS, from "The Second Coming"

~ My husband is prone to losing things: keys to the house, his driver's license, pens, even his wedding band. I first noticed this propensity on our honeymoon; when boarding our plane for home, he realized that he couldn't find our tickets. My favorite example of this ongoing, half-aggravating, half-comical tendency is that routinely, whenever ABC News wants to send him abroad on a breaking story, he can't find his passport. In his thirteen years at ABC, he has had to have three passports expedited by the American Embassy so that he could leave the next day on assignment.

Somehow during the fall and winter, he became hyper-organized. He endlessly researched the best doctors in the country for my condition, made appointments for me, arranged all of our travel plans to see these doctors, and managed to come home earlier from work than he had in years. Most meaningfully, he insisted on accompanying me to every one of my doctor's appointments. Ever the interviewer, he often asked more questions at these appointments than I did. He became the main caretaker of this family, an impossible position in which to put him, given the hours and demands of his career.

Yeats's poem "The Second Coming" likens chaos to a falconer losing control of his bird. The bird, flying in ever-widening circles, fails to keep its master at the center. Because of Eric's job constraints, I had always been the falconer, in charge of our domestic lives in the past. Now that I had abdicated all of my responsibilities, our family's center was not holding, even with Eric's heroic efforts.

Although I worried about what seemed an inevitable domestic crisis, I found myself increasingly incapable of handling even the smallest of tasks. Ostensibly in charge of our taxes, I neglected them. A missing K-1 form, which in prior years would have prompted me to barrage people with harassing phone calls, this year simply didn't get tracked down. I didn't bother returning e-mails or calls from my accountant and don't even remember if I ever signed our joint return.

So, too, bills stopped getting paid. Eric, in an effort to help, would fill out twenty checks at a stretch, but they too often bounced, sometimes because I would somehow forget to transfer money into our checking account, other times because my spending sprees had broken our budget. Invariably, these checks were to those individuals most responsible for keeping my family's lives intact: the tutor, singing teacher, piano teacher, and masseuse. Why couldn't the checks to Verizon, Time Warner, or Keyspan have ever been the ones to bounce instead? And I would find myself having to make abashed phone calls, attempting to explain in two hundred words or less that our family was struggling. Each individual was gracious about these mishaps, and for that I am both grateful and embarrassed.

Yet my memory lapses worsened, and I began forgetting things—my children's after-school activities, appointments, too often major events in my friends' lives (I didn't even check in with Leslie after her daughter underwent major surgery). Larger gaps began appearing in my memory. In one phone conversation with Amanda, she kept prodding me to remember a visit that she had apparently made only the day before. "Oh, Lynne, we were sitting on your bed, and I admired the flowers. I was picking Daisy up from a playdate with Lilly. Remember?" I remembered nothing. My brain, like a black hole, had sucked into its recesses any memory of her visit.

Our domestic life, frayed throughout the year, now began to unravel. Even the house started to rebel. All three bathrooms seemed intent on mutiny—faucets dripping, drains stopping up, and pipes losing hot water. By the end of the year, we didn't have a bathroom in the house that actually worked. Sometimes I watched the chaos unfold in detached indifference. Completely unable to muster the energy to get something to eat, let alone attend to our domestic turmoil, I would simply roll over to find a less excruciating position on the bed. More often, however, my memory lapses and lack of functionality terrified me. I would lie in bed obsessing about all of the loose ends but couldn't seem to keep them straight or handle more than a couple of responsibilities a day. It seemed a major victory just to pay one bill or to follow up on the phone with even one of my daily messages. As in Yeats's poem, chaos seemed close at hand, and it wasn't "slouching" but rather rushing toward our household.

Then, in a burst of energy, my mother took over. Dropping everything in her busy, successful life in St. Louis to be with me, sometimes for weeks at a stretch, she got our household back into shape by spring. She took on the role of surrogate mother to my children, honestly having more stamina and passion for them than I had at this juncture. She would watch Benjamin's piano lessons, play endless rounds of gin rummy with him, pick up Lilly every day from school, help her to navigate her nightly piles of creative but onerous homework, and even sit through her tennis lessons (the only parent/guardian/babysitter with enough fortitude to handle the absurdity of watching twenty giggling and inept girls repeatedly hit tennis balls into the net). Never had I been more grateful that my mother was so young and had so much energy (so young, in fact, that, on grandparents' day at her school, Lilly was utterly mortified when my mother quipped loudly in the stairwell, "What is this, grandparents' day or great-grandparents' day?").

When my mother periodically returned to St. Louis, Cora began caretaking me as much as the children. Exhausted but worried about me, Cora was selflessly loyal—helping me walk up the stairs, holding my hand, and wiping my forehead with cold compresses on bad pain days. I could offer in return only repeated and teary thank-yous, knowing that I was asking too much of her. Only with the help of these two women had apocalypse been averted, at least for the time being.

CHAPTER 17

The Furies

Abused, disappointed,
Raging I come—oh, shall come!—
And drip from my heart
A hurt on your soil, a contagion,
A culture, a canker:
Leafless and childless Revenge.
—AESCHYLUS, from *The Eumenides*

These words are uttered by one of the Furies; monstrous female arbiters of revenge in several Greek tragedies, they mercilessly hunt down those who have committed a crime until the criminal is driven by despair and exhaustion to suicide. In the weeks after surgery, I was initially patient, waiting for my pain to ebb, but, when it didn't, I eventually gave up and called upon the Furies, myself feeling like one of them.

Vengeance is mine! I would internally shriek but couldn't figure out where to direct this venom. Whom to blame? On whom to wreak my revenge? On Martin? I barely remembered the boy's name, let alone the boy himself. How could I fix him as the source of my woes? I could blame the original doctor who had allowed the halo brace to come off me before the bone had fused. Again, a shadowy figure on whom to focus such intense rage. How could he have known in the days before fusion surgery that the halo brace often did not work? Without the sophisticated X-rays and MRIs that exist today, the doctor probably didn't even see the nonfusion. So should I blame the brace itself, even though fusion surgery didn't exist twenty-two years ago? Or should I blame the X-ray machine? The newest pain management doctor? The neurosurgeon who had fused my neck, seemingly uselessly? I could blame myself for this mess. If only I hadn't pushed myself so hard. If only I hadn't started running. If only I had listened to the warning signals of my body more closely. My anger found this outlet difficult to maintain as well. Not even in my worst nightmare could I have imagined the full scale and scope of this predicament.

Without a target or an outlet for this rage, it simply festered, impotent. I railed. I fumed in a torrent of bitter hunger, complaint, and rebellion. I hated my new life, the pain, and the new limits of my body. I hated the shots, the surgery, and the many doctors who had confused and tormented me. I hated the sheer agony and loneliness. Jealous, brittle with envy, I resented anyone who still had an intact life. I wanted to dance on tables, to breathe freely, to play with my children, to have sex, to teach. My mind at this stage was utterly self-involved and myopic: me, me, me, me, I, I, I, I.

CHAPTER 18

Drugs

Little poppies, little hell flames,
Do you do no harm?

You flicker, I cannot touch you.
I put my hands among the flame. Nothing burns.

And it exhausts me to watch you
Flickering like that, wrinkly and clear red, like the skin of a mouth.

A mouth just bloodied.
Little bloody skirts!

There are fumes that I cannot touch.
Where are your opiates, your nauseous capsules?
—SYLVIA PLATH, from "Poppies in July"

Sylvia Plath, of course, killed herself—not by ingesting too many "nauseous capsules," but by sticking her head in the oven and breathing in its toxic fumes. I wasn't about to pull a Plath; I found the poppies instead.

Six weeks postsurgery, in the depth of a particularly bitter winter, I was popping Percocets around the clock; but they no longer worked. The pain felt worse than ever, so I began augmenting the Percocet with Dilaudid to combat the breakthrough spikes. This didn't help either. I kept calling my neurosurgeon, desperate and frustrated by his nonchalance toward my pain. He emphatically stated that, as he was out of state, it would be problematic to approve any more refills of narcotics. Because he remained hopeful that my pain was surgical and, therefore, only a temporary condition, he wasn't terribly concerned about my pain levels.

I had tried to avoid opioid painkillers throughout the fall, except when I was experiencing a real spike. Now I simply caved.

Opioid narcotics (so named because they are compounded from opium and opiumlike chemical substances) include, among others, oxycodone, OxyContin (the long-acting version of oxycodone), Dilaudid, Percocet, morphine, and methadone. They release chemicals in the spinal cord that block the body's pain receptors to the brain. Many of these drugs come from poppies. How could these flowers, the color of Hades' pomegranate seeds, Persephone's "mouth just bloodied," "little hell flames," produce such soporific effects? I have come to view the poppy as a particularly treacherous flower—by turns nefarious, lethal, and, contrarily, calming, numbing.

When to prescribe and how much to prescribe is controversial. In its June 4, 2007, issue, *Newsweek* reported that "almost 200 million opioid prescriptions get written in America each year. But 'widespread' does not mean 'effective' . . . In opioid trials, fewer than a third of patients on average report relief." A recent study, however, found that only 50 percent of chronic pain patients had received adequate supplies of painkillers. This is partly due to the low numbers of pain specialists in this country and partly due to the conservatism of most doctors, like my surgeon, who prefer patients to be off painkillers as soon as possible.

Finding myself more and more dependent on these pills was worrisome, as I had a terrible premonition that the surgery was not the cause of my pain, and that I would need a more long-term approach to combat my pain. I felt this way primarily because the postsurgical headache was in exactly the same place and at the same level of intensity as it had been prior to the surgery. The neurosurgeon and his nurse-practitioner both assured me that it was way too early to tell whether the spinal fusion had relieved the pain or not. He gave me three months as a minimum postsurgery to be patient and wait while the healing continued. In order to assist in this healing, he wanted me to take Valium. Muscle relaxants, he insisted, were more useful at this stage of the healing process than painkillers. Valium, though, simply put me to sleep for hours. When awake, I would still find myself in excruciating pain and felt that I needed real relief. Out of state, out of mind, out of surgery, out of mind, I thought bitterly and found myself yet another doctor in New York.

A kind and emphatic psychopharmacologist with an expertise in pain management, my new doctor agreed to refill my prescription of Percocet and increased the frequency of its dosages in an effort to halt the spikes. More coverage, in other words, to mask the pain more consistently. This worked, for about two weeks, and then the spikes began again. At this point, he took me off Percocet, explaining that, as happens with most painkillers, my body had developed a tolerance to the medication. He prescribed a different painkiller this time: methadone. Methadone, while used to treat pain, is more commonly known to help addicts withdraw from heroin. The body physiologically takes methadone in as heroin, but the mind feels no high. The doctor assured me that it was one of the most reliable and strongest painkillers on the market. I still had not fully recovered from the surgery, and it would provide much more dependable pain control in this temporary period of healing than the ups and downs I had experienced on Percocet.

He was, to his credit, partially correct. There were no longer any ups, or highs—just lows, and I began to fall. In the early days of taking methadone, I developed bloody slashes all over my body. I assumed that I had some new, horrible ailment. Shingles? Bedsores? Panicking, I showed up at the office of my brother-in-law David, a dermatologist, with no warning. I thrust my bloody arms and legs at him and shrieked, "What are these? They're all over my body." After hearing that I had recently started taking methadone, David calmly assured me that the bloody slashes were self-induced from scratching myself so hard; itchiness was one of the drug's side effects and would soon recede as my body adjusted to the medication. Repulsed by my self-mutilation, I swore not to scratch again and luckily didn't have to much longer, as the "itchies" did disappear.

Other more nefarious effects of this medication, however, did not recede; they just got worse the longer I was on the medication. Methadone, mixed with all the other crazy pills I was taking (including Neurontin and Valium), swirled me into a downward spiral. I became catatonic and could spend literally hours lolling away the time with a completely blank mind. More often, I passed out. Eric would come home to find me sound asleep in bed, my mouth hanging open, with Lilly propped next to me trying to do her homework or watching television. I would then get a second wind after the children were both asleep and would stay up until 4:00 a.m., watching reruns of stupid sitcoms and sleeping until noon. My schedule, nonconducive to children, husband, or friends, offered only deserted hours of quiet. Weary of noise, human contact, daylight, I wanted only silence, stillness, nighttime.

I became something of a nocturnal Arachne—and one indeed with a purpose. I took to crafty activities that required no neck movement, just hand-eye coordination. At first, I knitted, knitted, knitted. Scores of hats, legions of ill-fitting sweaters, scarves, baby clothes. Then the knitting began to strain my neck, so I switched to new diversions. My hands needed movement. So, I tried first embroidery (but the specificity of the patterns exacerbated my headache), then needlepoint (even worse for the headache—all those tiny little holes). Finally, I became hooked on jewelry making—nothing difficult, like wire wrapping— I didn't have the attention span anymore for such intricacies. Instead, I would simply bead, methodically dropping one pretty jewel after the next onto silk threads, creating longer and longer necklaces. When I decided that it was too taxing even to bother putting clasps on the ends, I created a lariat design, so that the necklace could just hang open and be tied around the neck. I found this excessively repetitive activity soothing, calming. I could do it for hours as I continued to float in a land without language, people, or purpose.

During this period, I did manage to get out of bed long

enough to have lunch with my friend Holly, whom since college I have called the voice of reason. All I remember about the lunch is that I cried a lot and that she wrote a list of "essentials" on a piece of computer paper that I was to repeat as my mantra. I remember gripping the paper the entire day, reading the words hypnotically. They seemed to hold some deep truth. Recently, I asked her what she had written on the paper, my memory having swallowed her words whole. She responded that she had been worried about me that day. I had ranted about tabloid queen Anna Nicole Smith's death, which the press initially reported as an overdose of methadone and other sedating drugs, a mixture similar to my own. Holly's words of wisdom on that precious piece of computer paper? Simply:

1. You are NOT Anna Nicole Smith.
2. You are going to get better.

Holly and I giggled over this one recently. Honestly, only a person on methadone could possibly think that these words held a talismanic power.

I have a picture with which to remember this phase. Taken after only eight weeks on methadone, the photograph shows me in bed. My face appears drawn with a sickly, white pallor. I am looking directly at the camera yet appear unfocused. My eyes look bruised, and my pupils shrunken. I am impossibly thin, cadaverous even, and my clothes hang on me. No question, I had transmogrified yet again, but not into bodacious Anna Nicole Smith, this time into one of the "heroin-chic" models of the 1990s, only shorter and older.

CHAPTER 19

Grief

It was the future you lived in,
as now you inhabit the past, and the two
have the same indeterminate sky,
brilliantly cloudless, the same
shifting walls between which
you place invented furniture . . .
    —LINDA PASTAN, from "Almost an Elegy"

An elegy, one of the most ancient of poetic genres, formally laments and commemorates a person who has died. I wasn't dead, however, so only an "almost" elegy could apply to me. I was living an almost life, a shade's life. Like Persephone, I too lived that winter in a liminal state, attenuated and stagnant, between the world of the living and the world of the dead.

After the neck brace was removed, I found the pain in my neck and head exactly the same as before the surgery. I felt tired of being brave and found it untenable to continue living in this present. So I began "inhabit[ing] the past," caressing the happy memories, lingering in past days of productivity, pining for the days of physical and intellectual pleasure. Craving joy, I was filled with grief, mourning my old life, unclear how to envision the future. So long had it been since my senses danced, I wondered whether I could even feel wonder anymore.

Why should anything have gone wrong with me? Why? Why should I have to endure this abyss? Since I had no interest in greater ontological or epistemological queries, I was solipsistic in my questioning. Overcome, I was dust to dust, ashes to ashes, a body spent, a soul impoverished. Linda Pastan so eloquently writes of this nearly expired life in the wake of pain and illness:

"I watch the shoreline of health / as it recedes in the distance. / I am nearly used up— / a lit match burning down / to my fingertips" ("Fever Dream").

Passion burned out first, replaced initially by desire, then longing. Longing figured as loss in my psyche. I felt longing for all that I had had in the past but that was now lost. Perhaps longing is the flip side of hope, as there exists an awareness, deep in the recesses of longing, of the impossibility of fulfilling the desire. One somehow knows that, no matter how extended or tireless an effort one makes to get back what one has lost, it is irretrievably gone.

I found that I most missed, even craved, having a body that felt desire, desiring, desirable. It made me itchy, antsy, wired, in a state of dis-ease, this longing, this crazy craving, but to fulfill my desire was equally crazy. A nurse taught me a fairly reliable technique for handling the nerve injections. Squeeze a small object in the palm of one's hand that has a hard edge, not sharp enough to cut the skin, but hard enough to elicit some pain. This pain acts as a distraction from the injection pain and makes the procedure more bearable. Eric and I tried to institute the opposite of this technique, substituting physical pleasure for pain. This replacement didn't work, however, as my body couldn't handle anything more than a foot massage or back scratch. Physical pleasure, while present with more intense forms of intimacy, also led to even more severe pain in my neck and head. And more longing.

As physical connectedness had become impossible with Eric, it had also become difficult with my children. I fiercely missed our former relationships. Maternal love, affection, and daily nurturing had always come naturally and easily to me. Only a year before, I had picked Lilly up, carried her about, and twirled her down the street. She had still snuggled into me every night, burrowing into my neck, legs piled on top of mine, in order to fall asleep. We routinely rubbed her tummy, which we had long ago decided was a magical oven, as it was always warmer than the rest of her body. So soft, so toasty, so delicious. She loved pressing the freckle right next to her belly button, her control mechanism for heating the tummy to an even higher temperature, and I would loudly exclaim, "It *is* hotter now. How can that be?!"

I didn't have a method of replicating that physical ease now, when every time she pounced on me, or tried to cuddle into my neck, waves of pain made it difficult to endure. Lilly's favorite chatting position had always been sitting atop my stomach; now her weight exacerbated the pain, and she would have to roll off me. I spent most of the day sleeping anyway, so I was even more physically unavailable.

Benjamin and I had also shared a physical closeness denied to so many of my friends with boys the same age. I had taught Benjamin how to dance—waltz and swing—but usually we simply turned on his favorite music and danced for the wild, sheer joy of it. He also had an ease about accepting affection, letting Eric and me throw an arm over his shoulder or kiss him good night. Since we could no longer dance together, I instead tried to be an audience of one to Benjamin's complicated African dance moves. Yet, when he would bound into my room with his indefatigable energy, the sheer volume of his voice and the banging of his feet would ratchet up my headache. In response to my repeated hushing, Benjamin simply receded. By the spring, Eric and Cora had to fill me in on the basic social relationships and his school life, and Benjamin began simply to check in on his way to his next activity, his next sports game, as if my knowing his whereabouts constituted a relationship with him.

I also missed the old me. Always bendy, flexible as a rubber band, I had loved stretching, yoga postures, feats of elasticity. After surgery, I was robotic. Unable to move my neck more than twenty degrees in any direction, I had to turn my whole body to look to the side. I couldn't look up or down and found walking down the stairs particularly treacherous. I had also acquired a rigid posture that permitted very little movement of my upper torso. This stance developed, perhaps, as a protective gesture, guarding my neck from making unnecessary movements that could spike the pain. This posture irked me, in particular; it was artless, awkward, graceless. Once again, my body had transformed, this time into an automaton.

Part of me knew that my grieving was unhealthy and that it could become a self-fulfilling prophecy; I had not let enough time pass. I might well find myself better over the next six months and able to resume my old life. Grief was, nevertheless, the place in which I mentally resided. In Elie Wiesel's words, "Despair is the question." I had not yet found an answer.

CHAPTER 20

Crest Falling

Good-by to the life I used to live,
And the world I used to know;
And kiss the hills for me, just once;
Now I am ready to go!
—EMILY DICKINSON, from "Farewell"

Wandering from one room of my house to the next, I seemed to have no purpose anymore. Always so busy when I had worked full-time, now I couldn't figure out what I was supposed to be doing with myself all day long. What was the point of my life? As February gave way to March, I began to fall further into a depression that not even a newly prescribed, strong antidepressant could abate. Crestfallen, I fantasized about crest falling; situated on the edge of a summit, I could simply go off. I had fallen off a cliff once before; I could certainly do it again.

I began thinking about suicide. To kill myself would also kill the pain, which no anesthesia had yet been able to do away with. No other means of escape seemed possible, and it was simply untenable to imagine that I could go on indefinitely enduring this level of pain. Nothing allayed my hopelessness. I was desolate and had become something of an Emily Dickinson in my reclusiveness and preoccupation with death and dying. Unfortunately, unlike Dickinson, I had no creative product to show for this morbidity. While Dickinson became a favorite role model, I perversely continued to fixate on Anna Nicole Smith as well, realizing that I resembled her more than anyone else. Instead of hundreds of poems tucked into my desk, like Dickinson, I had bottles upon bottles of pills shoved into my bathroom drawers.

This death triangle—Anna Nicole Smith, Dickinson, and me—
I knew was ridiculous, incongruous in the extreme. Yet, I rather
liked this unholy trinity, an orgy of death seekers, having given
up on hope.

Later that month, *People* magazine published the list of medications found in Anna Nicole Smith's body. Her autopsy revealed that she had died of "acute combined drug intoxication."
Eric brought the list home to show me, concerned because of
my own drug combinations. My worst fantasies about the odd
similarities between us became moot, however, upon reading the
list. The rumors had been inaccurate. She had not overdosed on
methadone, and our lists of medications were different:

Anna Nicole Smith	Me
chloral hydrate (Noctec)	
diphenhydramine (Benadryl)	Benadryl
clonazepam (Klonopin)	Klonopin
diazepam (Valium)	Valium (then current)
nordiazepam (metabolite)	
temazepam (metabolite)	
oxazepam 0.09	
lorazepam 22.0	lorazepam
	morphine
	methadone (then current)
	Ultracet
	tramadol
	oxycodone
	OxyContin
	Percocet
	Fioricet
	Darvocet
	Tylenol with codeine
	Ambien
	Lyrica (then current)
	Neurontin

Lidoderm
Skelaxin
baclofen
Robaxin
Zanaflex
prednisolone
naproxen
Zofran
Midrin
Pamelor
indomethacin
nortriptyline
isometheptene
Celebrex
Cymbalta
Lexapro (then current)
Wellbutrin
Keppra
magnesium sulfate
Thorazine
dihydroergotamine
Subutex

Of course, my list includes drugs spread out over the course of one year. She had taken many more drugs at higher dosages all at once—but still. The comparison suddenly foregrounded just how far gone I was. My therapist, like Eric, became focused on the mixtures of medications and insisted that as a matter of ethical responsibility she be permitted to speak to the doctor who had prescribed them. I will admit now that I took the danger of these mixtures as a positive. Like one of *Macbeth*'s witches, I could brew up a lovely little concoction and fall—this time, asleep—and never wake up. Painless and easy. I certainly had enough pills in my drawer to kill an elephant. I didn't need the Hemlock Society or *Final Exit* to assist in this suicide.

Initially, I didn't share these thoughts except for a couple of times—once to my poor mother, who must have been terrified. Outwardly, she kept her cool and just kept repeating, "You *are* going to get better, Lynne. You have to believe that. And you are doing great. We will get to the bottom of this. I just know we will." Easy for her to say, I thought. I felt like I really just couldn't go on much longer living in this kind of pain. I had become unmoored, floating useless out to sea. The pain was too all-consuming. I was enduring—but barely.

I also started asking myself, Why endure? For what? Was it the necessary "sacrifice" I had to make for the sake of my children? When could one stop sacrificing? I knew that Benjamin and Lilly needed me at least through high school—but, I began counting, that's nine more years for Lilly. I just didn't think I could hold on that long. The ghosts of the two suicidal poetesses Anne Sexton and Sylvia Plath, both mothers, were whispering too urgently: *Forsake the children, the responsibility, the morass of love. You deserve to be selfish. No one should simply have to endure.*

I had not been able to wrap my mind around the reality of my days. I felt that I was performing a vigil, waiting to get better so that I could resume my life; this stasis had seemed only temporary at first, but now appeared to offer no respite. My life was this waiting, and I had lost all hope of ever getting better. Louise Glück captures the unimaginable emptiness of this period in a heart-stopping passage: "A void / appears in the life. / A shock so deep, so terrible, / its force / levels the perceived world" ("Decade").

I did feel leveled, even though I knew that my perceptions were distorted. A couple of months later, I vocalized my dark thoughts more frequently, turning to various friends, some intimate, some less so, and received reactions from them that again shook my perceptions. One close friend referred to my confessions as "drastic-speak" and warned me to remember the power of words. If I verbalized a potential, I might thereby create that reality: but, I wondered, did that mean that I would remain trapped by that reality? Another friend interpreted my tell-all confession as a cry for help and wanted to stage an immediate intervention. Other friends traded war stories with me, each trying to outdo me with their own tales of misery. My sisters and mother allowed me to voice the worst without judgment or disapproval. It made me feel less alone with these thoughts, more capable of bearing this life. I also knew that I wasn't crying out for emotional or psychological help; I did want to be rescued, but rescued from my physical pain.

Eric and my therapist, however, had a different reaction altogether. After a flurry of concerned phone calls (both to each other and to me), they reassured themselves that I did not presently intend to off myself; but by sharing with them these dark fantasies, I had put myself in a vulnerable position. If I had present plans to hurt myself, my therapist had the right, even the ethical responsibility, to violate our patient-doctor confidentiality and hospitalize me. I went ballistic. I didn't need a sanitarium; I needed a cure for this pain. I held firm; she and Eric backed off, and I managed to avoid an asylum.

CHAPTER 21

Fallen

*I saw the best minds of my generation destroyed . . . suffering
Eastern sweats and Tangerian bone-grindings and migraines
of China under junk-withdrawal in Newark's bleak furnished
room. . . .*
—ALLEN GINSBERG, from "Howl"

I bottomed out in Florida during my children's spring vacation. I had just returned from my second follow-up appointment at the end of March and been pronounced by the surgeon "completely fused." Great news from a skeletal perspective, but my mother and I had pointedly questioned him about why I was still experiencing the same pain. Hadn't he told us that I would be out of pain once the bone had healed? We were so frustrated, so angry. He behaved genially toward us but somewhat indifferently. His work had been done, and now it was time for me to look elsewhere for help.

At the end of our meeting, he referred me to a pain center affiliated with his hospital for which he thought I would be a perfect candidate. My mother and I spent the afternoon listening to its chief administrators describe it: a monthlong outpatient program beginning in early morning and ending at 5:00 p.m., Monday through Friday. I could stay at a hotel near the center and have evenings to myself and even fly home on the weekends. The program offered group and individual therapy sessions; educational classes; hours of physical therapy a day; and IV medications the first week to help break the pain cycle. Although the doctors warned me that the program would demand much from me, both physically and mentally, they also thought that it would halt my downward spiral. I agreed to begin the program in ten days.

The plan newly invigorated me, and, at the encouragement of the doctors, I even decided to go off methadone so that I would be clean when starting the program. I met with my psychopharmacologist about how to withdraw from methadone safely. I was to take ten milligrams less every day for six days. Then I would be completely off of it before I began the program. He also assured me that at that pace I shouldn't have withdrawal complications. In anticipation of checking into the clinic (and how hard, in particular, that would be on me physically and Lilly emotionally), Eric and I decided to go with Lilly to Florida for her spring vacation. Benjamin was set to join my parents for the break. Lilly would, therefore, get lots of alone time with Mommy, which she badly needed, and I could get lots of R & R before the program began.

I'm a beach bum. I love the sound of the ocean, riding salty waves when the water is not too cold, and lying in the blaze of noon. For four days, although I still did no walking or moving, I lounged in the heat, soaking up sun, and watched Lilly swim for hours in the pool with her father. Lilly was a wonderful companion, and my favorite memories of those first days are of her reading aloud to me in the late afternoon shade, a book by our favorite children's author, Kate Dicamillo. I had also finished the methadone and was getting psychologically prepared to leave in a few days' time for the clinic.

A major twist in our plans occurred that Friday, after Eric spent hours on the phone doing further research on pain clinics. Apparently, they were all over the country. His research indicated that another neurological clinic had the best reputation for people with my problems, but it was an inpatient program that kept patients on an IV throughout their stay. Patients also had to share bedrooms. People considered this clinic the last resort, the final frontier, the place you went when all other options had failed. Patients apparently flew in from all over the world to go there. Eric called the clinic and spoke to the woman in charge of scheduling new patients. The outpatient facility could see me for an initial evaluation the following Thursday (four days into the other program). If they thought I was a candidate for their inpatient program, then I would wait for a bed to open in the hospital, which could be anywhere from twenty-four hours to a week. She said that they had approximately an 80 percent success rate of lowering patients' pain levels during the usually two-week-long hospital stay.

Just as suddenly as this new option occurred, however, I hit rock bottom. I called my mother and sister to discuss the two possibilities and found myself crying hysterically, uncontrollably, in the bathroom. Wailing, I kept repeating, "I don't know what to do. I'm freaking out! Which hospital should I go to? Or should I try one, and then, if I don't like it, switch and go to the other one on Thursday? Which? Which?" My sister and mother both tried to calm me down but found it impossible. Sobbing, I emerged from the bathroom only when Eric said that he had to make an urgent call for work. I forced myself to regroup when I saw Lilly lurking directly outside the bathroom door. Trying to avoid her seeing me cry, I pulled myself together and announced that I would take her outside for a swim.

There, as I stood by the edge of the pool, watching Lilly float about and do handstands, my headache spiked so quickly, so fiercely, that I thought I was going to throw up. The sun was strong, and I suddenly began sweating profusely. I then began shaking, violently. "Lil, Lil, you have to get out of the pool right now, honey, and we have to go upstairs," I managed to spit out. Confused, she actually listened, gathering our things, because I told her I couldn't carry anything. We got upstairs into the air-conditioned room, and I collapsed on the bed. My headache was, in Holly Golightly's words, in a "mean red" stage, and I started writhing on the bed. Then, suddenly freezing, I began shivering. I started putting on layers of clothing and pulled the blankets up over my head. Moaning from the pain, I began sweating again a few minutes later and threw the blankets off the bed.

Feverish, I thought that I had caught a terrible flu. Eric attributed the intensity of the headache to my having come off the pain medication. We decided to fly home early the next day instead of spending the weekend as originally planned. Lilly was not allowed to come into our room, a decision that seemed to intensify her anxiety, as she kept lurking at the doorway, trying to overhear our conversations. Eric kept whispering fiercely at me, "You have to hold it together. You are scaring her." Honestly, though, I couldn't. I felt like some satanic force had invaded my body. That night, my symptoms got worse. I was racked by a panic attack similar to the one I had had on the phone earlier that day. Yet this one, so taut, so intensified, so elongated, didn't go away the entire night. I began popping random pills in the bathroom. I must have been prescient about going off the methadone, because with a clean sweep, I had packed every medication on my shelf. I remember hurling myself onto Eric's lap at about 4:00 a.m. when he was sound asleep, squeezing his face, hysterically shrieking, "I think I'm dying. Do you think I'm OD'ing from popping all those pills? My God—I really am Anna Nicole Smith. Help me. What should I do?"

I don't know how we managed to get back to New York the next morning. Eric dumped all of our stuff into the suitcases and grimly escorted me through the lobby. The plane ride home was awful. I sat shivering under three airport blankets next to Lilly, incapable of uttering even a single word to her the entire three-hour flight. Stony faced, she sat quite still, looking small, vulnerable, watching a random movie the airplane was showing. When we got off the plane, Eric rushed me in a wheelchair through the airport and put me in a car service to take me home. He and Lilly stayed behind to collect the baggage.

The moment I got home, now Saturday afternoon, I called my psychopharmacologist, whom I had not called from Florida;

I left a message at his office, hoping that he checked his machine on the weekends. I then called the newest of my pain doctors. I had only seen him a couple of times. He was famous, and I had waited months to get an appointment with him, hoping that he would have a new diagnosis or some creative ideas about how to treat me. He had merely reconfirmed the prevailing diagnoses and advised a new litany of medications. When he had seen me right before I had started going off methadone, he had seemed alarmed at that decision, saying that I would have no protection from the pain. He wanted me to begin seeing him more often and, in addition to muscle relaxants and anti-inflammatories prescribed by his neurologist, wanted to put me back on Neurontin, this time at a higher dosage, and another narcotic called oxymorphone—again I was to fall into morphine? I had left his office frustrated. I certainly wasn't going to take a step backward and begin taking medications again that had had such powerful side effects and hadn't even worked anyway. In such desperate shape now, I nevertheless had him paged.

I waited hours for the doctors to call back, shivering in bed, thinking that they could help me. Saturday evening, my new doctor, enraged that I had bothered him on a weekend, finally did call back. The call lasted all of one minute. I quickly explained my symptoms and asked him what I should do. He informed me that he didn't have my chart at home, and if I couldn't wait until Monday to see him in his office as I properly should, then there was nothing he could do for me, and I should just go to an emergency room. He then promptly hung up.

Alarmed, Eric began doing what he does best—investigating, researching, making phone calls—getting to the bottom of a story. I continued to huddle in bed, sicker than I had felt the whole year. Lilly was again exiled from my room, and, no fool, she listened. I spent those hours obsessing that I had permanently traumatized her. Late Saturday night, Eric calmly came into the room, informing me that I was experiencing methadone withdrawal. My body had not been able to tolerate going off the medicine so quickly. He then recited a partial list of typical withdrawal reactions: anxiety attacks, mood swings, headaches, increased pain, restlessness, insomnia, chills, sweats, and cold and hot flashes.

"That's exactly what's wrong with me," I responded. To myself, I thought that I resembled a drug addict I had watched in a documentary years earlier in which he had freaked out, writhing and crying on the floor from trying to go off of heroin cold turkey.

"So," Eric pronounced, "you need to take some methadone right now."

That was a problem. I didn't have any more, just an unfilled prescription from the psychopharmacologist that luckily I hadn't thrown away. Eric called every pharmacy in New York open that late on a Saturday night. They all had the same answer. "That is a controlled substance that we do not keep in the pharmacy. It has to be ordered." Panicking, he actually drove up to a methadone center in Harlem that night, hoping that they would take pity on him and give him a couple of pills to get me through the night. That attempt, desperate, yes, I know, also failed.

A true junkie now, I spent another sleepless night, this time obsessing about how my husband, now my pusher, would score for me the next day, given that it was April 8, Easter Sunday. Every pharmacy would undoubtedly be closed. We would not hunt for Easter eggs this year—only for drugs. No chocolate bunnies, sugar-coated sweets, or baskets of jelly beans for me— I just wanted methadone. Months after this incident, it became one of my favorite gallows-humor tall tales—going through heroin withdrawal in Miami. Getting through that night, however, was grim, at best. And, only later, would I learn just how dangerous these few days had been. In retrospect, I should have listened to the doctor and gone to the emergency room.

Miraculously, Eric managed to get my prescription filled on Easter Sunday. Sloan-Kettering, a New York hospital famous for treating cancer patients (many of whom take methadone for pain relief), had an in-house pharmacy. They willingly filled my prescription. By this time, I had also spoken to my psychopharmacologist, who agreed that I should go back on the methadone until I could withdraw from it in a more controlled setting. Eerily, within an hour of taking my first twenty milligrams of methadone, all of the withdrawal symptoms vanished as quickly as they had started.

So the decision of which clinic to go to the next week crystallized for me in a millisecond. I was scared at how my body had rebelled and instinctively knew then that I needed to be in a hospital under twenty-four-hour surveillance. The outpatient program would not offer me round-the-clock care, and the idea of being alone in such a fragile condition in a city where I knew no one terrified me. Now restabilized on the methadone, I would wait in New York and regather my strength, which after three sleepless nights and all of that physical and psychological drama had suffered a setback. I would fly out to the clinic on Thursday. One of the nurses on call advised me to taper off just thirty milligrams of the methadone before they saw me on Thursday but not to stop taking it altogether. The doctors would provide medications at the hospital that would make the withdrawal symptoms more bearable.

PART II

A Paradise Within

. . . only add
Deeds to thy knowledge answerable, add faith,
Add virtue, patience, temperance, add love . . .
*   then wilt thou not be loath*
To leave this Paradise, but shall possess
A paradise within thee, happier far.
   —JOHN MILTON, from *Paradise Lost*

CHAPTER 22

April

April is the cruellest month, breeding
Lilacs out of the dead land, mixing
Memory and desire. . . .
    —T. S. Eliot, from "The Waste Land"

Both Anglo-American literary traditions—beginning with Chaucer's *Canterbury Tales*—and Christian typology associate the month of April with hope and resurrection. Classical Greek mythology also associates springtime, the time of Persephone's return to earth, with rebirth. Yet the beginning of modernist poet T. S. Eliot's "The Waste Land" twists these traditions. The beginning of April for me, first going through withdrawal on Easter and then persevering through my first week at the hospital, looked like I was heading into a modernist spring, perhaps not cruel, but certainly not—at first—rejuvenating. As the month progressed, in conformity with literary tradition, as well as just coincidentally, my mind began slowly to thaw, relax, and bloom. Spring brought me, like Persephone, back to earth.

My initial consultation at the outpatient facility of the headache clinic confirmed the obvious—their inpatient program at the hospital would serve my needs better than the outpatient program. Waiting for a bed to open and getting preauthorization from my primary insurance carrier, too, proved uncontroversial. Within only forty-eight hours of our consultation, Eric and I arrived at the hospital for my admission.

It was early evening. Eric's plan was to get me settled, help me to unpack, and then catch the last flight back to New York so that he could be home in time to put Benjamin and Lilly to bed. A nurse showed me to my new home; a generic-looking hospital room and antiseptic bathroom greeted me. The only peculiarity was a dingy curtain pulled across the middle of the room to separate the two beds. My roommate wandered in a few moments later, grabbed a sweater, and without introducing herself left the room. I heard her in the hallway chatting with a group of other patients who were all going to dinner together. I suddenly felt like the most unpopular kid in junior high. How was I going to get through these weeks alone? I felt disoriented and couldn't believe that my life had actually come to this. Nine months into this ordeal, I was in yet another hospital, still in pain, still unsure of my diagnosis, still with no answers. Thousands of miles away from home, my children, my life, I felt like I had been incarcerated for some awful crime.

I began reading the schedule posted on my bulletin board. IV medications would begin at 5:00 a.m. Doctors would make rounds soon thereafter, followed by breakfast at 7:00 a.m. Mandatory classes were conducted all morning, followed by lunch at 11:30 a.m. and further classes in the afternoon. IV medications were again administered at 2:00, followed by dinner at 5:30 p.m. Final doses of IV medications would be administered at 10:00 p.m. Preventative oral medications, also administered three times a day, were interspersed in between the IVs. Abortive medications, used in the event of a pain spike, would be administered on an as-needed basis.

I am and have ever been a confirmed night owl. I never, ever get up before 8:30 a.m., and even that time is pushing it for me. One year, at the mandatory parent-teacher conference, I heard little about how Benjamin was faring. Instead, the teacher spent the twenty minutes reprimanding me, because he always arrived late to school. Since that incident, my children have technically arrived at school on time. Somehow they manage in the mornings without me. My son walks with his friends to school at 8:15 a.m., never having even seen me awake; and, before this year, I would wake up at the last possible minute to walk Lilly to school by 9:00 a.m. The running joke for years with my neighbor Jane as she saw me clutching my coffee cup, stumbling sleepy eyed down the block to get Lilly to school, was that she (and probably every other mother in my neighborhood) had already been up for hours, gotten the kids to school, and managed to play an hour of tennis. A hospital schedule, beginning at 5:00 a.m., I kept thinking, could not possibly work for me.

At that point, a rather stern nurse wheeled an enormous scale into the room to weigh me, pronouncing that these mandatory weigh-ins would be conducted twice a week. Self-conscious about my emaciated form, I balked and for the next few weeks would try to avoid these awkward invasions of my privacy— when, of course, I had no privacy. "One hundred five pounds," she grumbled.

She then glanced at my mega-bags of M&M's, my Starbucks coffee grinds, and my hot pot for brewing them, already laid out on the bedside table. She announced firmly, even accusatorily, "Chocolate, coffee, and any form of caffeine are forbidden here. They are migraine triggers. Also, that hot pot could start a fire. It cannot stay." I can't utter a sentence until I have had my first perfectly brewed cup of Starbucks in the morning. What she was suggesting violated my very sense of propriety. This was supposed to be a head clinic—no caffeine for me would mean an even bigger headache! And, since Easter, I had developed a preternatural need for chocolate (I would later learn that craving sweets is another lesser-known symptom of methadone withdrawal). "But," I stammered, "I'm not a migraine patient." "That's irrelevant," she countered. "Many other patients are and will not be able to tolerate the smells alone."

Following on that nurse's heels, another nurse appeared who took my vital signs and then wanted to begin an IV right away. I asked if I could have a few moments alone with my husband first and then went ballistic. "I am not staying here. You realize that, right? This is just too grim. I can't do it."

Eric, ever calm, ever able to read my moods, said, "I knew that you were going to try bolting. I even have a bet going with your sisters. Don't worry. I'm not going back tonight. I'll stay until tomorrow and smuggle you in a cup of Starbucks." Feeling alienated, already homesick, I dreaded Eric's leaving the next day. I couldn't imagine how I would be able to stay here without his support, without any of my usual creature comforts, and without knowing anyone. I had no interest in making new friends or bonding with fellow patients like my roommate. What could I possibly have in common with all of these sundry people? I decided that I would just stay in my room and not talk to anyone.

After settling me in, Eric accompanied me on a tour of the hospital as I dragged my rolling IV behind me. The main common room, used both for classes and entertainment, had a television, rows of chairs, and several games and puzzles stacked against the walls. My roommate and her clique, sitting around a long wooden table, were engrossed in a game of cards and barely looked up when we entered. In the basement, the nurse showed me how to work the industrial-looking washer and dryer. I won't have to use those machines, at least, I thought, having had the foresight to pack enough clothing for a fourteen-day stay. Only later, as my stay dragged on well past the fourteen-day mark, would I, of necessity, have to grapple with those machines (which turned all of my delicate, pastel-colored underwear gray in the process). In the linen closet, the nurse showed me where I could find sheets, blankets, and towels for bathing. No luxury hotel, this hospital—not even a Motel 6. I would be making my own bed, doing my laundry, and, apparently, drying myself with tiny yellowing towels the size of my hand towels at home. It will take four towels just to dry my body, I thought, and another four for all of my hair (which, after a year without a haircut, was heading toward my waist). The nurse further instructed me that when I wanted to take a shower, I would need a nurse to unhook my IV first and then wrap the exposed needle in my vein with layers of cellophane and tape, so that the needle wouldn't get wet. Beginning to cry, I must have seemed so pathetic that the nurse took pity on me and said that I could finish my orientation the next day.

After Eric left, and I was lying on my bed, trying to figure out how I was going to sleep on my side with the IV needle on the underside of my wrist, my roommate reappeared. She did finally introduce herself and informed me that she was leaving first thing in the morning. So that meant yet another stranger with whom to contend by the next afternoon.

My first week at the hospital, I was bewildered, extremely sedated by the medications, and hampered by my IV line. I couldn't understand why other new patients were tethered to twenty-four-hour lines for only three days and the rest of their stay hooked up to an IV only three times a day for a short period. I, conversely, was attached to the IV for eight full days and nights. I never figured out quite why the doctor wanted me to be hooked up all the time. Was it because I was underweight and needed additional fluids or nutrients? Because I was detoxing from methadone? Because they were trying stronger medications on me? My mother thought it odd that I never found out the reason. My passivity and lack of interest were not in character, as usually I wanted to know every detail about a situation and would ask incessant (or, to my mother at times, pestering) questions. Yet I found myself in those early days with little energy to take an active interest in my care. Whatever the reason for the IV, it continued to be a nuisance.

I also found the daily schedule difficult to navigate; I would struggle awake at the crack of dawn when, at morning rounds, the room would suddenly fill with nurses, doctors, physician's assistants, and psychologists, a swarm of bees who would flow in and out so quickly that, at first, I had trouble being alert enough at these meetings to get my questions answered. As the days progressed, I learned to write the questions down, pop up in the bed, and quickly fire them out, before the swarm buzzed away. I also got special permission from my doctor to have a cup of regular coffee in the morning. Nothing is worse than hospital coffee, not even airplane coffee, but it was better than no coffee at all. I would roam the halls in my pajamas, a monomaniac, searching for pots of coffee, which in our wing didn't exist. Though I accepted the rigor of the hospital's Betty Ford clinic–esque, narcotics-free policy, I simply refused to give up my addiction to caffeine.

I went to every class I could during my stay at the hospital but realized with chagrin that, during the initial week, I wasn't able to follow even the subjects of the lectures, let alone their principal messages. As the weeks progressed, I found myself inadvertently reattending some of the lectures, not even aware that I had heard the lecture before. Only upon returning to my room to place the handouts in a folder would I realize that I already had copies of the same handouts. I felt like an Alzheimer's patient.

Certain aspects of the hospital would remain intolerable throughout my stay—the unappetizing food, the excessively cold climate (particularly daunting given my withdrawal chills), and the ever-more-difficult efforts to find workable veins in my arms for the IVs. IV lines needed to be changed every three days, but my veins seemed to give out after only two days. I would lie motionless as nurses dug around in my veins, sometimes in five different places before finding a vein that could handle the lines. These nurses were fascinating to observe, reminding me of baseball players with their odd superstitions and rituals. If a nurse couldn't get a vein after three tries, then she would back off, sometimes muttering "Bad karma" under her breath, and have another nurse take over. At 5:00 a.m., however, these belabored efforts were nasty indeed.

The early days of my stay in the hospital were mostly marked by methadone withdrawal. I learned that methadone is even more addictive than heroin and that my symptoms could go on for several weeks. I became used to putting on three sweaters and, minutes later, stripping them off. These chills and sweats, I originally thought, were my most pronounced symptoms now that I was having my withdrawal managed by several medications. My doctor soon corrected this assumption, providing me with significantly more information about my drug use. Many of my headaches could be the result of overuse of narcotics, what he called rebound headaches. Further, even though I was now off methadone, it still had a half-life in my body for the next three months. My pain spikes could be a response to drug withdrawal. Worse, after almost a year on and off various opioid narcotics, my brain chemistry had been altered.

Because of my brain's lack of efficiency, I was not highly receptive to the many IV and oral medications that the doctors were trying on me to bring down my pain levels. The hope was that these IV medications could break the pain cycle, that is, the repetitive loop of nerve signals to my brain. Like the hamster that can't stop running on a treadmill, my body was unable to stop obsessively sending alarms to my brain. So inured to the help of opioids, my brain had lost its natural ability to receive and process pain signals properly. My nervous system had, in a sense, short-circuited, bombarding my brain with pain signals that could be false. Further, pain begets pain. One needs to stop the pain loop long enough for the brain to rewire itself and to begin processing pain accurately. The process of "rebooting" my brain could take as long as six months. As one of the hospital's doctors explained, "We are only at stage one in your recovery."

My doctors also thought that my jitteriness, anxiety, and depression, which in these early days at the hospital were manifested mainly by uncontrolled crying jags (during classes, meals, alone in my room, on the telephone), were caused by the chemical alterations to the brain. The hospital's psychologist explained that methadone had interfered with my brain's normal serotonin receptor and dopamine levels, both necessary for a healthy emotional life. Further, withdrawal from methadone exacerbates feelings of not only anxiety and mood swings, which I already knew from Eric's research, but also depression.

Recent surveys attest to the inadequacy of opioid narcotics to address chronic pain over the long haul. They too often do not alleviate the pain, as I found, or they do so only temporarily. As one's body begins adjusting and developing a tolerance to the medications, one is forced either to take more of the painkiller or to switch to a different (usually stronger) painkiller. As with all medications, there are also side effects, ones that I found unbearable—dizziness, loopiness, extreme sedation, to name just a few. Worse, these medications, in my experience, destroy the mind, the soul, the spirit. Catatonic for months on these drugs, I had lost the will to fight, to get out of bed, even to live. While pain doctors try in good faith to relieve suffering through the use of medications (and, in some instances, only painkillers can do the job), another school of pain doctors, like those at the hospital, think that the risks outweigh the benefits of relying on them for chronic pain relief and that they can, in some instances, actually make the pain worse. My own experience turned me into something of a die-hard Addict Anonymous. At the hospital, I was determined to "kick the habit" and vowed to find new solutions to address my ongoing pain.

CHAPTER 23

Hope

No more be mentioned then of violence
Against ourselves, and wilful barrenness,
That cuts us off from hope, and savours only
Rancour and pride, impatience and despite. . . .
—JOHN MILTON, from *Paradise Lost*

⌒◯⌒ How does one regain hope when it has splintered and then shattered? The shards fallen in every direction. Some swept up and thrown in the garbage. Other pieces hidden, between floorboards, behind furniture, wedged into cracks. Another piece walked off after lodging in someone's foot.

Regaining hope would be my most difficult task at the hospital. As always, my brain needed to hitch itself to a fictional narrative to accomplish this mission. The myth of Isis and Osiris, one of Milton's favorites, provided that place of intersection. The plotline of the myth is simple. Seth, Osiris's brother, kills Osiris, in order to take the throne. After killing Osiris, Seth hacks Osiris's body into fourteen separate parts and scatters them throughout Egypt. Isis, Osiris's beloved wife, searches for and finds thirteen of these parts and, with her magic, brings him back to life long enough to conceive their son Horus (who eventually takes back the throne and revenges his father's death).

The complexity of the myth resides in its multitudinous interpretations. It was traditionally interpreted as symbolizing the cycles of birth, death, and rebirth, and its celebration took place, unsurprisingly, in springtime. Milton preferred to interpret the myth as symbolizing the search for truth, which since the fall from grace had been scattered and would only be made whole again at the Second Coming. I overlaid my own interpretation onto the myth. Osiris came to represent hope to me. My hope had been shattered by the events of the fall and winter, but its pieces had not been destroyed. They were just missing in action, separated from their necessary other parts. The task was to reconstruct hope's fragile form, perhaps never completely, but at least partially. The hospital, as my stay continued, came to represent Isis, as it methodically, diligently, tirelessly began helping me with the difficult process of piecing my broken hope back together.

A creature of habit, I adjusted to the rhythms and routines of the hospital by the end of the first week. I began to handle the constant monitoring of my vital signs, pain levels, and emotional state fairly well, after watching my roommate's blood pressure drop dangerously low in reaction to one of the medications. The negative aspects of the hospital became tolerable, particularly in light of how much good the experience was having on me. One unanticipated benefit of the hospital stay was that it allowed me the luxury of focusing only on getting better. Domestic, work, and social responsibilities ceased to exist, and I had few distractions or even much outside contact; my only task was to attend to my fragile mind and body. In the isolated setting of the hospital, I began to strive again.

My neurologists were my lifeline during this period. One significant event occurred in the second week of my stay that felt like a breakthrough. I had been obsessing about the fusion surgery and whether I should have listened to the doctors who had told me that it was unnecessary. I had also read a recent study that pronounced that spinal fusion surgery "had no acceptable evidence to support it." I worried that the surgery had not only failed to help my pain levels but also made the situation in my neck worse—more pain, more muscle spasms, and less mobility. I finally asked my neurologist his opinion at morning rounds. He said that he would have to review the hospital records and MRIs. The next morning, he met with me and emphatically stated that the fusion surgery had been "necessary" and "life saving." The MRI showed that the instability had been so near the brain stem that it had needed to be stabilized. All of the injections attempted before the surgery (that is, the twenty-one shots of the fall) had been destined not to work due to the continuing instability.

Somehow, hearing this information from a by now trusted doctor had an immediate effect on my mental state. It put to rest many of my most nagging anxieties and fears. I felt my depression begin to lift and my mood reinforced by the neurologist's morning rounds, at which he cajoled, cheered, and heartened me. He insisted that he had great hope for my recovery and that, while it might take a year, I would indeed get significantly better. His optimism, humanity, and sheer energy countered the previous months of despair and resignation; I found myself listening to him, believing with him that I had a chance.

I also give credit for my changing mental state to the work I was doing with the cognitive-behavioral psychologist assigned to me. Early on, I just cried and cried, sputtering out incoherent thoughts that ranged from "I'm worried I will never get better" to "I feel guilty that I can't take care of my children the way I used to" to "I'm worried I'll never teach again." Cognitive-behavioral psychotherapy focuses on the relationships between thoughts, feelings, and behavior and has the potential over time to cause the patient to change her thinking patterns and adopt new thinking circuits. The therapist spent a great deal of time breaking down my distorted thoughts, likening my reasoning to that of a person sitting by the side of the road who, rather than calling for help, just sits there agonizing over how and why the car broke down. "Doesn't get the driver back on the road, does it?" she asked with a smile.

I responded particularly well to her efforts to reorient my negative thought processes, as her method also got the analytical side of my brain working again. She gave me daily "homework," asking me, for example, to write out as many "dysfunctional" thoughts as I could, determine why they were dysfunctional, and then rewrite them to be more realistic. For example, my abiding terror was: "I will never get better." This was dysfunctional, because it represents "all-or-nothing," "catastrophic," and "fortune-telling" thinking. My revision: "It is too early to know how much better I am going to get. I need to give this more time." What could be better for the perpetual student and academic in me than the three-prong process of writing, interpreting, and revising?

The therapist's homework was the first time in almost a year that I had written anything. Just holding the pen to paper felt reassuringly familiar, like muscle memory, when one's body remembers how to do a cartwheel, ride a bike, or, in my case, a plié. I began seeing the therapist nearly daily for private sessions, so thrilled finally to have a new way of approaching my pain. I pounced on the homework, in particular, finding that it was girding me round and slowly dissipating much of my anxiety and depression.

Another important aspect of the hospital's treatment plan for me included several more diagnostic shots—an epidural, more occipital nerve blocks on both sides of my neck, and aggressive temporary blocks on several nerves from C2 through C5 on both sides (seventeen shots in all). I was relieved that the nerve shots could all be handled in one procedure and, further, that I could be asleep throughout it. This alone was a radical departure from the fall, in which I had endured so many useless hours of additional pain having shots administered one at a time with no accompanying anesthetic. I considered this new pain anesthesiologist a cowboy in his aggressive approach to treating my pain. The epidural had no tangible effect, but the other shots seemed to bring down my pain quite substantially for a couple of hours. Pleased, the doctor hoped that he had "hit a bull's-eye." The more permanent RF ablations could not be done while I was an inpatient at the hospital. We, therefore, scheduled them for after my departure.

Hope is amorphous—fragile, tenuous, so easily lost. Many different components, both external and internal, worked together to begin bringing hope back into my life. The multidisciplinary approach of the hospital in no small part contributed to hope's return. To those chronic pain patients who are struggling alone without hope, I find myself wanting to help them search far and wide, like Isis, to grasp at all the little fragments and shards that only together can bring about a change of heart.

CHAPTER 24

Patience

When I consider how my light is spent,
Ere half my days, in this dark world and wide,
And that one talent which is death to hide
Lodged with me useless, though my soul more bent
To serve therewith my Maker, and present
My true account, lest He returning chide,
Doth God exact day-labour, light denied?
I fondly ask; but Patience, to prevent
That murmur, soon replies, God doth not need
Either man's work or his own gifts. Who best
Bear His mild yoke, they serve Him best. His state
Is kingly. Thousands at His bidding speed
And post o'er land and ocean without rest:
They also serve who only stand and wait.
  —JOHN MILTON, "Sonnet XIX"

I miss teaching "Sonnet XIX." Usually devot-
ing a whole class period to it, so that we can linger there, savoring every technical and structural nuance, I work with students
to understand the poem on both personal and formal levels.
Milton wrote the poem about the onset of his blindness; when
he relates that he has lost his light, he refers both to physical
light and to spiritual light, the light of God. Because he has gone
blind, he is railing against God, questioning his fate and thereby
his faith. He uses the Parable of the Talents to accomplish this
message. Like the worker who buried his gold coin (or "talent")
in the earth, not using it to beget further talents, he had been
punished by his Maker and flung into outer darkness. Milton
sees his "talent" as his ability to write. Yet by questioning the
mysterious ways of God in the first seven lines of the poem, he
has blasphemed, even restaged the fall from grace. His question-

ing is as dangerous as Adam and Eve eating from the Tree of Knowledge. It indicates a loss of faith in God.

The final six lines of the poem doctrinally answer the sonnet's principal question: what does God want from us? Simple, straightforward, these lines read like prose, and the didactic message is clear to all. God wants our faith. Omnipotent, he doesn't need our earthly achievements or require our work. Omniscient, he alone knows what our true talent is supposed to be. Milton must wait—patiently—for his true purpose to be unveiled by God in its proper time. And then, in the extraordinary last three lines of the poem, vision returns to the poet. In a poem wholly without visual description up until this point, Milton triumphantly, majestically, ends with a true physical as well as spiritual vision.

"Sonnet XIX" became my talisman at the hospital, a concrete symbol of all that I cherished when I found myself so far from home. I took to whispering it to myself, deriving comfort from the recitation of this familiar, long-loved, and much-studied poem. Sometimes a line would follow me about for the day, haunting my thoughts, in the same way that a song can get stuck in one's head. In particular, the phrase "dark world and wide" resonated with me. I felt that I had suddenly been thrust into such a world—overwhelming, alien, and hostile. Then the phrase "his state is kingly" would rush to the fore, and I would find myself buoyed and stronger. I would then find myself repeating the last line of the poem, myself striving to be patient, to be at peace. Rarely have I so deeply internalized a poem, and once it had taken up residence within me, it began expanding in my mind. It settled both my mind and body, and I took to breathing the poem, literally, during relaxation exercises, an activity new to me and encouraged by the hospital.

The doctors instructed us that daily biofeedback and relaxation exercises are tools for coping with chronic pain. Relaxation reduces stress, allows contracted muscles to let go, changes one's breathing, blood flow, and skin temperature, and breaks up abnormal physiological processes. Thus, regularly practicing relaxation exercises has the potential to change the brain's neuronal connections, even the structure and function of the brain over time, and thereby bring one's pain down to a lower level. The hospital supplied us with relaxation tapes, biofeedback training, and yoga instruction. I began listening to the tapes while at the hospital, and relaxation exercises became one of my regular practices. I honestly don't know whether they have ever brought my pain down to a lower threshold, but they are an assuredly better way of getting through the grueling hours when the pain spikes than just staring at the ceiling as I used to do. Sometimes, though, I find it difficult to stop my brain long enough to be in and of the moment; when I have such difficulty, I try to be kind to myself, reasoning that a relaxed New Yorker is an oxymoron anyway.

My favorite relaxation exercise in the hospital (and to this day, whenever it is hot enough) is to lie flat on my back outside in the heat of the sun. All of that warmth penetrating every pore of my body, I begin breathing in through my nose and out through my mouth. I then concentrate on my toes, consciously willing them to relax. I move my way methodically up my body all the way to my head, relaxing the different muscles in my body individually. I learned this technique from one of the CDs by Alan Lake, "Relaxation and Pain Management Strategies," given to us at the hospital; but then I diverge from his routine and begin to recite Milton's "Sonnet XIX" over and over again in my head.

There, at the hospital, in the middle of nowhere, for perhaps the first time, I found myself connecting with Milton's work at a deep emotional level, feeling that this poem was talking to me in ways I had never before heard. I, too, had been railing—not against God per se, but at my fate. Feeling sorry for myself for months, nearly done in by such vicious pain, I had also found myself in spiritual darkness. I realized later that this phase of my hospital stay was important transitionally. It opened up my mind to new ways of thinking about my physical problems and my life. Perhaps, I began to think, if I can no longer teach Milton's poetry, I will still be OK. Perhaps I may never finish my book on Milton, but I will nevertheless have a more profound tie to his work than I ever had before when only my rational, analytical mind was engaged with his poetry. Perhaps words would be available to me again and still provide the sustenance that they always had before. Perhaps a little bit of hope and a little bit of patience in the future were what I needed. I still must remind myself of these lessons daily, and "Sonnet XIX" remains my favorite mantra and easiest access to these lessons.

CHAPTER 25

Courage

Fifty years without limbs, or in an iron
lung, is that possible? I lose
courage but courage is not lost.
　　　—GEOFFREY HILL, from *The Triumph of Love*

꧁⁓ I had always found the literature of morality somewhat distasteful. For so many centuries, literary critics, beginning with Aristotle, argued that literature must not only bring pleasure but also teach something of relevance to its reader. The reader, ideally, should learn to profit by example, and this process usually occurs by first admiring and then wanting to emulate a worthy character. Epic heroes, in particular, display those virtues important at any given time to the dominant culture. One such virtue, courage, has consistently appeared in literary works across time and place—from classical Greek to Renaissance epics, from eighteenth-century to nineteenth-century novels—and yet presents itself in many different guises. For example, martial daring on the battlefield is emphasized in classical Greek epics, while spiritual strength is privileged in Christian Renaissance epics.

I do not consider myself a particularly brave woman, never have, and during this period I found myself, in Hill's words, "lose courage" all too often; but at the hospital, among many of the other patients, "courage [was] not lost," and, for perhaps the first time in my life, I found myself surrounded on all sides by individuals who displayed true valor. Every patient in the hospital had his or her own unique story of hardship and coping to tell. Some of these narratives were more heartbreaking than others, yet all of the patients at the hospital grappled with their demons and displayed acts of sheer determination during their stays.

People's stories, for all of our individual idiosyncrasies, shared a common theme: we felt that our struggles with pain had severely compromised our work and family lives in ways that healthy people cannot and do not understand. It was a relief to be among the like-bodied and like-minded. We had all been worn away, pillaged by pain. There was no need to explain myself, my level of misery, suffering, exhaustion, or body loathing; everyone there was living the same crippled and crippling existence.

After spending months feeling that my life was too difficult to bear, and that everyone I knew had it better, I now faced a startling shift of perspective. I was one of the luckier ones, mercifully spared many of the ancillary hardships endured by patients. While I had managed to get a leave of absence without much difficulty and had job security for which only tenured professors and judges can hope, the vast majority of patients at the hospital needed to continue working for economic reasons—long-term disability insurance and social security disability did not provide patients with adequate economic stability. Forced to continue at their jobs to support themselves and their families, most patients faced further hardship, as they found themselves vulnerable to the wrath of uncompromising employers. One woman, who worked for a government agency, described how, if she were to make a mistake on an official document, it would be deemed a criminal offense. Unsupportive of her chronic pain, her employer had punished her for her condition, assigning her to work the graveyard shift. Sitting alone in an empty governmental building, imprisoned in her physical suffering, she had had to endure the additional terror of thinking that, if she didn't accurately do her job, she could literally go to prison.

Patients saved their harshest vilifications neither for their employers nor for the government, however, but rather for medical insurance companies. All of the patients were having their hospital stays covered by private medical insurance; very few people in this country would be able to handle the costs of such an extended hospital stay without significant assistance from insurance. Yet nearly every one of our insurance carriers only partially covered our medical expenses. We complained about the seemingly arbitrary limits placed so often on our reimbursements for medical expenses. The carrier would inexplicably label an expense beyond the "reasonable" amount charged for a particular appointment or procedure and limit the reimbursement accordingly. Other times, for no apparent reason, the carrier would deny coverage altogether.

One young man had the worst of all chronic migraines—the dreaded cluster, which he explained felt like someone was gouging his eye with a burning poker. This headache is one of the most unbearable to endure and the cause of higher incidents of suicide than any other; nonetheless, this young man approached his condition with a consistently gentle and good-natured affability. He had had to drop out of high school, and then within five days of his arrival, he had to drop out of the hospital, as the family's insurance carrier refused to cover any further days of inpatient care. The insurance carrier's decision not to cover the young man's stay felt criminal, particularly as the hospital seemed the only recourse available to him. How many chronic pain sufferers were out there with no insurance and so had to fend for themselves with all of the attendant financial burdens?

Patients related fending for themselves in other ways as well. In several classes, patients exposed their families' indifference to their suffering, describing how a parent, sibling, spouse, or child rarely called, showed support, or offered help. Their loneliness was as palpable as their grief over these rejections. Privy to such personal information, I found myself thinking so much about my own marriage, feeling profoundly beholden to Eric. His sensitivity and loyalty contrasted quite starkly with the responses of so many of the other spouses.

The most extreme example of spousal neglect took place

within the confines of the hospital itself. One of the women most consistently compassionate to other patients revealed in class through teary punctuations how her husband as much as her pain had been unrelenting. Insensitive to her suffering, he had bordered on abusive—coming into their bedroom where she lay in the dark silence of pain only to turn on all the lights and begin questioning her about what was for dinner. Needless to say, she hadn't been to the grocery store or even out of bed that day. He insisted that she get up, prepare gourmet meals for his clients, conduct herself totally normally, and continue running the household with no help. The day she calmly underwent one of the more gory procedures used at the hospital—a nerve block into the eyelid—she came back to her room to find her husband waiting for her there with divorce papers.

There were, conversely, as many stories of devoted spouses, parents, lovers, and caretakers. Often family members accompanied patients to the lectures. In some classes, family members had an opportunity to speak, and at such times, they earnestly voiced their devotion to their suffering spouse or child. Selfless in their loyalty, determined to provide whatever emotional support they could, these caretakers demonstrated compassion that I found nearly as compelling as the patients' own courage.

In the wake of such loyalty, many patients, including myself, were plagued by guilt over how we had destroyed not only our lives but also our families' lives. One woman explained during a class that her migraines left her face half paralyzed. Her mouth and eye drooping, she sometimes slurred her speech. Sighing, she described how one of her youngest children had unconsciously taken to imitating her facial droop and speech patterns. She felt guilty and helpless; I found myself awed by her stamina. How had she, in such pain, managed to care for five children? She must have been doing something right for her child to want to emulate her.

A young girl who had already withstood three brain surgeries had a chronic condition of leaking brain stem fluid. Her head pain, therefore, was just a minor symptom of a more catastrophic illness that did not seem to have a cure. She was extremely quiet, subdued throughout her time at the hospital. I admired how she never complained. Indeed, I only heard her story as hearsay from other patients. Always lapidary, she kept her dignity in the face of a terrible reality. Most impressively, her parents stayed at her side all the time, attending every class and meal with her, mobilized to stay resolute, no matter what, for the sake of their daughter. Only a few times, when not in the company of their daughter, did I see their composure crack to reveal a glimpse of the personal toll such support was taking on them.

We all felt a toll; self-pity, as well as guilt, pierced each person's courage at some point in the hospital stay. One girl with an inoperable, although benign, brain tumor had been forced to drop out of school because of her head pain. She sighed one evening over dinner, admitting that it was the night of her senior prom, her "last chance" to go to a prom, as she had been too sick to go to the others. This led to an outbreak of sorrow as another woman began weeping at the table. She had missed her son's graduation from college that same day. I, too, was depressed that night, having missed my sister Jeanne's fortieth birthday party. There we all found ourselves, sequestered in this odd location, missing the great moments of our lives. Searching for a solution to our pain and fortified by constant reinforcement of our tenuous selves in the hospital came at a price: exile.

Patients at the hospital not only shared banishment but also shared certain patterns of behavior. While I am no anthropologist, I did find it striking to observe how this enclosed community developed its own innate character and bonding rituals. The hospital's hermetic environment produced two distinctly different personalities in its patients even in the time that I was there. I initially found myself a member of a group of middle-aged women, motherly types, as am I. Our group shared similar activities (like knitting), interests (many of us were in the field of education), and often took yoga classes and ate our meals together. We were a panoply of odd illnesses—a fibromyalgia patient, a survivor of a brain embolism initially misdiagnosed as a thunderbolt migraine, a car accident victim who had had her skull stapled back together, a daily migraine sufferer for the past eight years, and another neck fracture patient.

Eventually, we even had our own leader, although during the first week in the program, we rarely saw her. Exhausted and continually vomiting from her withdrawal from a cocktail of eight different medications, she did not attend classes or meals. I would see her briefly being wheeled down the hall looking drawn and devoid of personality. After getting through the worst of her withdrawal, she unexpectedly blossomed into the resident den mother of our group. Her naturally gregarious personality reawakened; she began socializing, finding us at mealtimes, laughing heartily. One day, she went to the gift shop and bought all sorts of homey items—quilts, pillows, and decorative objects—to brighten up her room and invited us over for a social visit.

All exploring different treatment and medication options, we kept up a steady conversation, swapping anecdotes, advice, and mutual commiseration. My initial instinct to sequester myself in my room and not meet anybody, I found, led to the opposite reality. I have never bonded with such a small group of individuals as quickly or deeply before (perhaps camp as a girl is the closest parallel). The hospital experience, so set off from our usual support networks and asking so much of us both physically and mentally, created a unique environment in which to develop deep ties.

I, therefore, watched with a mixture of panic, sadness, and exaltation as one by one the individual members of my group began departing—often leaving behind small gifts (a knitted scarf, a bouquet of flowers, a sweet note)—each and every one of them better off than before their stay. After the first two weeks of my stay ended, I found myself alone as a new crowd succeeded my original group, and I began playing the part of a welcoming crew to all of the newcomers.

This new crowd was a little younger, a little wilder, a little more tenacious. Rebelling against the strictures of the hospital, they took to going out after dinner on walks that took them technically two hundred yards off the premises. Their "illegal" forays were to an ice-cream shop next door to the hospital. Their sleeves rolled down to cover their IV lines, they would order decadent ice-cream cones and sit together late into the evenings chatting or watching dark comedies. Their defiant escapes to the ice-cream store reminded me of the patients in *One Flew Over the Cuckoo's Nest* when they made their big run for it, and I dubbed these patients "inmates on the lam."

I had my soul mates, at any rate, people with whom I hope to stay in touch for the long haul. We all had something in common that led to our initial bonding. My closest friend, Jude, was my roommate for most of my stay at the hospital. We were so compatible that I could have lived with her for months longer. Enduring what we did together, we became true comrades-in-arms. Intimate with each other's daily struggles and problems, we prepped each other for morning rounds; we listened in on each other's conversations with the doctors, sometimes simply acting as another set of ears to interpret the doctor's answers, other times calling out a question that the other had forgotten.

I also became close with the other neck fracture patient at the hospital. A beautiful Southern belle with both charm and self-deprecating humor, she revealed at dinner one night that, like me, she had broken her neck twenty years earlier. After enduring a decade of chronic pain without any relief from traditional medications, she had turned to alcohol to dull her pain, only to get into a car accident and break another vertebra in her neck. Finally clean, she was at the hospital to combat the belated effects of these two accidents.

My other closest bond was with the only other methadone addict at the hospital at that time. I joked with him that he at least looked like a heroin addict—a twenty-something drummer in a rock band, he was tattooed and pierced and had a punk haircut. Two junkies, we spent hours commiserating over our withdrawal symptoms and pain levels together, and I still keep up my most consistent stream of e-mail correspondence with him.

Meeting other people with similar problems had a healing effect upon me. I no longer felt so alone or unique. I realized that others shared my most intimate problems and had found their lives equally impacted by pain. The hospital catapulted me out of my seclusion, and I thereafter felt differently toward my situation. I began to learn a bit of compassion, and it permanently shattered my previously ingrained patterns of narcissism. More invested than before with the other patients, I also found that I had profited by the example of these patients, willing myself to be stalwart and not give in to feelings of despair. I also vowed to find a support group for chronic pain patients once getting back to New York. I realized that being surrounded by a community with whom I had something in common was critical to my emotional well-being. Now that I had both "world enough, and time," I would search out these relationships.

CHAPTER 26

Reclaiming Life

I want what everybody wants,
that's how I know I'm still

breathing: deep mix, rapture
and longing. . . .
　　　—MARK DOTY, from "Mercy on Broadway"

In the second week of the program, my father visited for the day. So relieved to see a beloved face, I nearly wept just at the sight of him. In his usual quiet manner, he offered much-needed familial support. He had brought a gift for me, a copy of the video *Slow Dance*, created for Jeanne by her brother-in-law and close friend for her birthday. They had shown the video at her birthday party, which I had missed a few days earlier. The video begins with a song gently crooning "Take your time / Take a breath," and the screen shows a ballerina, gliding on her toe shoes, twirling leisurely, languorously, in layers of gauzy pink netting. The nearly hypnotic song and turning ballerina suggest aesthetic pleasure, beauty, physical connectedness, the slowing of time. Such a perfect reminder for so many, like my sister—raising children, working full-time, racing from commitment to commitment, by turns harried, fulfilled, and exhausted. The piece is achingly beautiful and, yet, so inappropriate thematically for me, whose own life had not merely slowed but screeched to a deadening halt, that I cried. Again. For the thousandth time that year. Grieving that part of me that had been lost more than twenty years ago, I was also longing for my reinvented self, who had improvised a full and engaged life that after nearly a year had seemingly vanished.

How could I reinvent myself yet again? And what would this reinvented self even look like? Jeanne's video reminded me that ballet had provided an answer to such questions after my car accident. Part of my crying was the belief that it could not provide the answer this time. How could it? My pain was so intense that I could barely get out of the hospital bed. And so my sister's birthday video, the close-ups on those beloved toe shoes, haunted me throughout my hospital stay, and for months after, as I struggled to find some way to regain my life this time.

Later that afternoon, I was forced to consider this issue again. My father accompanied me to a class that I had initially wanted to skip. Known as particularly tough, the class provided patients with better coping skills for living with chronic pain. My father insisted that we go. The teacher, a pragmatist, emphasized that we would all likely have to endure pain for the rest of our lives. This straightforward statement set me on a crying jag. My father quietly handed me Kleenex and then held my hand or rubbed my leg—only making me cry the harder. I was both touched by these comforting gestures and frightened by the teacher's bleak prognosis. At one point, the teacher suggested that we should work hard to make sure that pain did not become our lives and that we "should not let our lives pass us by."

This message has had an enduring effect upon me. Thinking back on that first year, particularly the frenzied search for new doctors, I realized that I had let life pass me by. Our family had spent all of our collective energy, time, and effort searching more and more frantically for a medical cure for my condition. A mock-epic quest, if ever there was one. In the process, I had stopped living anything even resembling a life.

There is a critical episode in Edmund Spenser's *The Faerie Queene*, a romance-epic from the sixteenth century, in which the knight Calidore temporarily abandons his quest to hang up his helmet and shield, to dally with his lady love Pastorella, and to watch the Graces dance. Arguably the penultimate moment of vision in the poem, the scene may well detail the true ethos of the romance-epic hero: while remaining dedicated to his quest, he must nevertheless make sure to balance his life with moments of rejuvenation, love, and aesthetic pleasure.

Even though I often taught this poem, I had neglected to grasp, or even notice, this critical moral lesson. I had utterly failed to profit by Calidore's heroic example. I look back on all of my earlier complaints of feeling lonely and isolated and must admit that these emotions stemmed in large part from my own behavior. Languishing in bed, waiting for my pain to disappear altogether, I had routinely canceled plans with friends. I declined every single invitation to a family event, dinner, or party that year, often sending Eric alone to enjoy himself. So terrified of spiking my pain, I had become a wallflower, watching the dance but not participating in it, and thereby missed out on those life moments that would have most succored me. The only event that I managed to attend that whole year was a funeral. The celebrations of life—birthdays, anniversaries, weddings, holiday get-togethers, congratulatory parties, book parties—went unattended.

I also wasted any opportunity to have learned or grown that year. There were so many lectures occurring in New York, some by eminent scholars in my field and outstanding writers, and, after circling the announcement, originally intending to go, I would find myself on the day of the talk still in bed. Always so particular about my children's regular attendance at museums and at gallery openings at both my father's and sister's galleries, I look back now to realize that I attended only one opening the entire year.

My own habits intensified my isolation in other ways as well. My tenaciously static condition had become so boring, so tedious, to me that I worried that other people must feel the same way. In response, I became increasingly hermetic, sealing myself off further from the world outside of my bedroom. I regularly screened phone calls in order to avoid more discussions about my physical condition. My family loves action—control freaks, every last one of them. Stagnation, lack of progress, and the loss of a consecutive narrative were all unbearable to them. I could only offer the broken-record response, "What more is there to say? I feel exactly the same today as yesterday." I became so disgusted with having the same discussion again and again that I found it easier simply to evade such conversations and so began a strategy of avoidance.

I remember one evening when I went out to dinner with a friend of twenty-five years. We hadn't seen each other in months, and I missed her. I spent the entire evening conversing with her about the details of her life—asking for and accordingly receiving a blow-by-blow account of her work status, details about her child and parenting tactics, and the intimacies of her marriage. I did this, in part, because I was so desperate to feel "normal" again and to escape yet another circular discussion that inevitably ended up back on the topic of my neck. At my bidding, she launched into an extended story of her husband's twenty-four hours in the ICU and how traumatic this had been for them both. At this point, I could barely restrain myself from shrieking, *A twenty-four-hour event with no lasting effects or physical consequences of any kind? Are you kidding me?* The three-hour dinner ended, and I hadn't alluded even once to the fact that I was in the middle of a crisis. She left the dinner knowing absolutely nothing about it. An opportunity to share with a friend not only her struggles but also my own could have brought us closer. Instead, I left the dinner feeling even more alone. Somehow, wanting to feel like my old self, I had lost the rhythm and reciprocal give-and-take of human interactions.

Life is different with chronic pain. It often is absurdly, categorically abnormal. How to reestablish normalcy—of activities, interests, and relationships? Where to start? Being a mere voyeur of the lives of others, living vicariously through my children's, my husband's, and my friends' lives, would no longer be enough. I had to figure out how to step back into my life once I returned to New York. After so many months of letting my life pass me by, I had no idea how to reclaim my life; I just knew that I had to do so.

CHAPTER 27

Faith

Two roads diverged in a yellow wood,
And sorry I could not travel both
And be one traveler, long I stood
And looked down one as far as I could
To where it bent in the undergrowth;

Then took the other, as just as fair,
And having perhaps the better claim,
Because it was grassy and wanted wear;
Though as for that the passing there
Had worn them really about the same,

And both that morning equally lay
In leaves no step had trodden black.
Oh, I kept the first for another day!
Yet knowing how way leads on to way,
I doubted if I should ever come back.

I shall be telling this with a sigh
Somewhere ages and ages hence:
Two roads diverged in a wood, and I—
I took the one less traveled by,
And that has made all the difference.
  —ROBERT FROST, "The Road Not Taken"

At the beginning of my third week in the hospital, a fellow patient asked whether I would be willing to attend a short nondenominational service in the hospital's chapel. Generally indifferent to organized religion, I define myself as culturally Jewish but spiritually agnostic. I, nevertheless, agreed to attend the service. When I arrived, the group of patients, led by one of the patient's husbands, a minister, all held hands and began praying out loud. I was not close friends with any of the people in this group and barely knew some of their names.

Yet it turned out that these individuals had organized the prayer session in advance especially for me. Their words were spontaneous, simple, uttered with gravity and clarity. They had noted that I was struggling. A truism at this stage, medications had not worked well to combat my pain levels, and the doctor had not yet determined whether I could have RF ablations because of the titanium wiring in my neck. They asked God to help give me faith in the future, belief in his inscrutable ways, and to find a way for me through the wilderness. In Milton's words written to explain why he wrote *Paradise Lost*, these kind individuals were "justifying the ways of God" to me. I was deeply moved by their gesture and openly wept.

Later that day, one of the men from the prayer session gave me a copy of a prayer written by Catholic theologian Thomas Merton: "I have no idea where I am going. I do not see the road ahead of me. I cannot know for certain where it will end . . . But I believe that the desire to please You does, in fact, please You . . . And I know that if I do this You will lead me by the right road though I may know nothing about it."

That evening, my newest (third and final) roommate, a devout Baptist from Texas, offered me a passage from the Old Testament (sensitive and respectful of my Jewish upbringing, she said that she had avoided the New Testament). Intending to read me another passage, she accidentally gave me Isaiah 43:18–19: "Remember not the events of the past, the things of long ago consider not; See, I am doing something new! Now it springs forth, do you not perceive it? In the desert I make a way, in the wasteland, rivers." Although not the passage that she had initially wanted, we both agreed that this passage was all the more appropriate. The metaphor of the road and a new journey again, as in the prayer session and Merton passage, predominated as the spiritual lesson. She interpreted this incident as one of God's little miracles, letting us know that he is always looking over and out for us.

And I honestly saw more miracles in my time at the hospital

than I had ever seen in my life. Patients who arrived in the worst possible shape physically, some having endured even decades of chronic head and neck pain, were leaving with no pain or radically reduced pain. Often, the doctors properly diagnosed a patient who had gone sometimes for years with the wrong diagnosis. Migraine sufferers, in particular, found proper medications to control their symptoms. People with neck injuries, like me, often responded to the aggressive injection treatments. Patients practically sang out the "Hallelujah Chorus" in the hallways on a daily basis.

Nevertheless, I must admit that my foray into religion proper, becoming a born-again Christian, let alone much of a Jew, was short-lived. Of all the religions, I did find myself leaning for a time toward Catholicism. I loved all of the saints, finding it particularly appealing that I could light a candle and pray to Ursicinus of Saint-Ursanne, patron saint of stiff necks; Ubald of Gubbio, patron saint of neuralgia and migraines; Madron, patron saint of pain relief; and Teresa of Avila and Bibiana, both patron saints of headaches. Teresa of Avila's symbols were a heart, an arrow, and a book; I, needless to say, found myself immediately drawn to her. Nevertheless, I still did not feel that spirituality would be the answer for me. In Anne Sexton's words, "I can't. Need is not quite belief" ("With Mercy for the Greedy").

For so many of the patients at the hospital, having spiritual faith, praying, and actively participating in their religious communities offered them a kind of peace and strength to bear their pain that was not available to me. A poll conducted by Stanford University Medical Center indicates that 58 percent of American patients look to prayer to help ameliorate their pain and that, for about half of these patients, prayer works as well for pain relief as prescription medications. While prayer would not be my "road," in Merton's words, it stirred and inspired me to think that we could each find our own "way."

I began to reflect further on faith. I was reminded of Milton's

own disastrous forays into organized religion, and finally his re-
bellious declaration that he was "a Church of one," refusing the
strictures and limitations of any particular sect. So what, where,
then, was my church? Was I too "a Church of one"? If I subscribed to any religion, or if my soul had any faith at all, then it
was in the power of art—to heal, to uplift, and to provide hope.
Aesthetic pleasure had always held a privileged, sacred place in
my life. A room of Mark Rothkos, *A Midsummer Night's Dream* in
thirty Indian dialects, the Bolshoi Ballet performing *The Pharaoh's
Daughter*, and, most centrally, "dreaming by the book," in Elaine
Scarry's words, gave me faith. To me, poetry had never represented a mere luxury, a genteel activity in which one participated
while sipping tea from a Limoges teacup; rather it represented a
means of survival. Most of my mothering had been to instill this
faith in the hearts and minds of my children. I insisted upon
nightly, nonnegotiable hours of reading and, since they were
toddlers, had read poems out loud to them by Gerard Manley
Hopkins, for example, or John Keats, thematically only nonsense
to them, simply for their sensory sense, their symphonic sense.

And that is how an odd little convergence occurred—not a
miracle—but a wonderful poetic similitude to the prayers of my
fellow patients. My family came to visit the day after the prayer
session, and I proudly took them on the "woodland walk" that
weaved through the hospital grounds. After so many months of
near sedentary status, I hoped that this exercise would be noted
as significant by my family. We got to the beginning of the walk
where two roads, in Frost's words, literally "diverged." One of
peat and dirt led directly into the woodland walk. The other,
cement, led to a nearby gas station. My lovely Lilly, the city
slicker, Brooklyn born and raised, headed directly down the cement road. We all howled with laughter, explaining to her that
she was meant to go into the woods. "That's why it's called the
*wood*land walk," her brother shouted, for emphasis.

Unimpressive in early spring, this walk offered up by way of
visual interest a few rotting logs, some trees beginning to bud, a

few purple violets, and one mangy-looking deer in the distance. Within minutes of this ill-fated effort to enjoy our natural surroundings, Lilly began to sneeze and her eyes to water. Wailing, "I'm allergic to this walk," she began to run in the opposite direction. We again erupted in laughter both at her silliness and at the ill-suitedness of our urban family to handle even fifteen minutes in the woods. We happily turned back toward the concrete sidewalk of the hospital parking lot. As Lilly's allergic symptoms receded, I began reciting Robert Frost's "The Road Not Taken," joking with Lilly that she indeed desired to take the "one less traveled."

After this incident, I again found myself thinking about roads, journeys, and finding my way. I had spent the year feeling lost, identifying only with literary characters who found themselves in hell searching for a way back to earth. Each of us wayfarers on an archetypal journey. I realized with utmost clarity that while spiritual faith would be "the road not taken," I would perhaps find other options to lead me home and provide me with the strength and sustenance I so sorely needed. Perhaps our family would find a way to carve out a road into the future—it just might not be the one well traveled. Maybe for our family, as for Robert Frost, this would also make "all the difference."

When we got back to the hospital, I looked at Lilly and asked, "Do you know how far we walked?" She shook her head, confused. "This is how far it takes to get to your school and back. Maybe, just maybe, Mommy is getting a little better and will be able to take you to school now and again when I get home," I responded. The first day I arrived home from the hospital, I did indeed walk Lilly to school—for perhaps the third time all year. When Lilly came home from school that day, gripping her homework, she thrust it at me with a grin. Her assignment for the week was to memorize Robert Frost's "The Road Not Taken."

CHAPTER 28

Where Is Demeter?

Yes, this year you feel
at a loss, there is no Demeter
to whom to return

if for a moment you saw
yourself as Persephone.
It is she, Demeter, has gone
down to the dark.
        —DENISE LEVERTOV, from "Talking to Oneself"

What if all of this time, I had been misreading the myth of Persephone? Maybe I wasn't like Persephone at all but rather like Demeter, no longer the girl in need of maternal protection but instead the mother whose duty it was to protect her daughter. As in Levertov's poem, I had both misinterpreted and abandoned my role and duty. I had "gone down to the dark," but descending into the underworld was an unforgivable act of selfishness for a mother. I had swapped our proper roles. In an effort to stave off perpetuating such maternal neglect, I agreed to have Lilly visit me again.

Eric and I had made the mistake of telling Lilly that my hospital stay would last at most fourteen days, never imagining that I would remain in the hospital for more than three weeks. After her first visit to the hospital, Lilly began to have trouble. By day nineteen, she had hit her limit. I was flooded with weepy phone messages on my cell phone. Up until then, I had rarely taken phone calls while in the hospital. Now I found myself having lengthy conversations with Lilly several times a day. She missed me terribly and insisted that we allow her to skip school and stay with me until my return home. Realizing that we were at fault for having mismanaged her expectations, we reasoned that perhaps another visit would ground her, allay some of her anxieties. On this trip, however, despite all of our good intentions, there was no pacifying of Lilly's worries, let alone a faith-confirming mini-miracle as had occurred at her last visit.

Because Eric had to work, my sister Jackie agreed to bring Lilly to the hospital, an unprecedented act of loyalty, as it required Jackie to stay in a children's room of the neighboring Holiday Inn and share a bunk bed with Lilly. Jackie graciously embarked on this adventure, even letting Lilly call the top bunk. The morning went beautifully; they arrived straight from the airport, and we were all in high spirits. Lilly insisted on acting as a tour guide and showed Jackie all around the hospital. Lilly was also eager to meet my new roommate and see some of the people who had been so nice to her on her first visit. Capitalizing on our success, we took Jackie first on the woodland walk and then meandered down to a small children's playground on the edge of the hospital's grounds. At the infamous ice-cream shop next to the playground, Lilly got to choose anything she wanted; she settled on a dish of mint-chip ice cream with rainbow sprinkles. I had not walked so far or so long since my stay began. I had always declined going to the ice-cream shop with the gang of "inmates on the lam," because I worried it would overly tax my body. For Lilly, though, I would have tried to climb Mount Everest. Feeling guilty that I had left her for so long, I wanted so much to spoil her with maternal nurturing.

The walk proved an unmitigated failure, spiking my pain as high as it had been my entire stay. We got back to my room, and I just couldn't. Couldn't. Do anything. Lilly wanted to cuddle, to chat, to play with my hair, but my body went under. I needed medication and sleep to regroup. Jackie, who notices everything, soon suggested that she and Lilly go on a "special" activity and return in time for dinner. So relieved, I went into a deep state of pass-out, only struggling awake when they returned. Jackie, the dear heart, had taken Lilly on what sounded like an exhausting outing, replete with a trip to a teddy bear factory (where Jackie bought Lilly the biggest bear they had) and to an enormous indoor playground.

Lilly did not seem fazed by my nap, probably inured to this need. She returned to the hospital quite happy, excited to show me her new teddy bear. I, on the other hand, had been shocked by my body's meltdown. I suddenly remembered my body's vulnerability and how little energy, strength, or stamina I actually had. Even after all of the medications tried in the hospital, the injections, the IV, the coping strategies, and the psychological help, my pain levels remained the same. I would be leaving the hospital mentally stronger, but in no better shape physically.

Settling Lilly in my bed after dinner to watch a rerun of *I Dream of Jeannie*, Jackie and I, under the pretext of finding Lilly a soda, escaped to a small kitchen stocked with supplies at the end of the hallway. This was the first moment that Jackie and I had managed to be alone together, and with such a sympathetic audience, I wept, long and hard. I told Jackie that I didn't know what I was going to do. How could I return home? Insulated within the confines of the hospital, I had found my pain levels more under control, but I had also spent half of each day asleep. How could I resume my sedentary lifestyle upon returning home? To continue to behave as an invalid even after the hospital stay would feel like failure.

At this moment, one of the gang of "inmates" peeked in; she wanted me to know that she had found my daughter roaming the hallway looking for me. She and the other inmates would hang out with her until I calmed down. A public spectacle, I had devolved in clear view of all the other patients. Worried, Jackie and I immediately went to find Lilly. Seeing her surrounded by strangers, trying hard to be a big girl and a good sport, I bled. She seemed more fragile, more in need of protection, than she ever had in the past. I knew that feeling lost, unable to find me, in a scary place with sick people, perhaps even having heard me cry, had wrenched her. The disparity between what Lilly and I both wanted—normalcy, the return of Mother, of health, of shared joys—and this perpetual dystopia had never appeared starker.

Jackie and Lilly left the next morning after first coming to say good-bye. Lilly seemed withdrawn, somewhat withholding. The trip, hyped as girl time, replete with Mommy and Auntie bonding, had failed. It neither allayed her anxiety nor brought her happiness. The aftershocks of this latest trauma would take months to surface, but I worried right away that upon my return home I would continue to disappoint Lilly's expectations.

CHAPTER 29

Pacing

I have measured out my life with coffee spoons.
—T. S. ELIOT, from "The Love Song of J. Alfred Prufrock"

Eliot's protagonist in "The Love Song of J. Alfred Prufrock" spends much of the poem talking about se- ducing a girl, but, trapped by his insecurity, indecision, and wa- verings, he never acts. Self-critical, he likens his overly cautious behavior to "measur[ing] out [his] life with coffee spoons," sug- gesting that this tendency has led to a life of banality.

Such a description received a decidedly different interpreta- tion at the clinic in a lecture devoted to teaching patients how better to pace themselves; the teacher referred to an article by Christine Miserandino entitled "But You Don't Look Sick: The Spoon Theory" in which the author describes the difference be- tween a healthy person and one coping with pain (or any sick- ness) in a parable that also involved measuring out one's life with coffee spoons. The healthy person has been given an enormous number of spoons (that is, enough energy and stamina to ac- complish necessary chores and work and still have enough "spoons" left over to enjoy the evening). The person in pain, on the other hand, has only a limited number of spoons and thus has to make tough choices and sacrifices in planning the day. The teacher stressed that learning when to say no, slow down, or take a break was critical in the life of a person dealing with chronic daily pain and, further, that pacing oneself could lead to an en- hanced quality of life.

The teacher also emphasized that we must take responsibility for our pain. We should identify and try to avoid our personal pain triggers. For migraine patients, this could mean any number of foods, smells, atmospheric conditions, caffeine, even inadequate sleep. For me, the triggers always involved movement that would jostle or inordinately move my neck, particularly running (the bang-bang-bang of my footsteps on the street) and bumpy car rides (a necessary evil in New York City where every street is riddled with potholes).

I found this simple lesson crucial upon my reentry into New York life. Upon my departure from the hospital, after a three-and-a-half-week stay, I was given detailed instructions on which preventative medications to take every day and which medications I should use as abortives (once the pain had spiked). These medications, none of which were opioid narcotics, ran the gamut from withdrawal medications to anti-inflammatories to muscle relaxants. All in all, I felt that the clinic had literally saved me, as I was leaving the hospital with a radically improved mental state. Physically, however, I continued to struggle and, from my perspective, had not yet found any pain relief. I remained hopeful, nevertheless, as I would imminently return to the clinic for the RF ablations and another follow-up with my doctors.

Contending with the pain levels continued to be my principal occupation upon my return. I began to realize how much benefit I had received from my old narcotics and missed that hazy, floaty existence. I also realized that the IV medications given at the hospital had worked more efficiently than the various oral medications prescribed at my discharge. My new medications did not provide the same floor to the pain that now without the narcotics had a new edge and sharpness to it. On the first day home, in order to avoid any moment of weakness, psychological or physical, I threw away all of the pain medications that had littered my shelves (Dilaudid, oxymorphone, OxyContin, oxycodone, Darvocet, Percocet, and tramadol). While I could have made a small fortune on the black market, I was mostly eager just to have all of those "killers" out of the house. Privy to no temptations, I would continue to abstain from overusing opioids.

The concept of pacing, however, proved easier in the abstract than in the reality of our domestic lives. The pile of invitations and announcements about my children's end-of-year performances, recitals, and events greeted me upon my return. My calendar quickly filled up just with the "command performances." I also wanted so much to reconnect with friends that, overly ambitious on only my second day back, I accepted an invitation to a charity luncheon in Manhattan to which I went every year, thanks to my friend Juju, who always bought a table. Excited, I put on one of my retail-therapy relics that had been hanging unworn in my closet. At the lunch, embraced by several close friends, I felt like it was, in Heather's words, my "coming-out party." At dessert, however, my pain spiked with a vengeance, and I exited the lunch without even a proper good-bye or thank-you to Juju. Lying down in the backseat of a taxicab, feeling frustrated and angry, I groused to myself, "My body can't even handle a simple lunch."

Hours later, when the spike still had not ebbed, I grabbed a syringe and a vial of Toradol, my strongest abortive medication, and headed to my in-laws' medical office, only two blocks away. My sister-in-law Rella kindly saw me unannounced and gave me the shot. After a two-hour nap, I woke to find that the shot had gotten my spike under control.

Pacing myself, measuring out my days with coffee spoons, became my new reality. Particularly at first, I rebelled against the strictures of my body and overdid things—always with the enormous cost of an angry spike. Pacing myself was initially frustrating, and I felt marooned in a house locked from the outside. Eventually I learned to store up an adequate supply of stamina so that I could splurge on the extra luxuries. Pacing thereby allowed me to have sometimes only small window boxes, other times expansive meadows, of normalcy, and I found myself regaining some of my independence and autonomy.

CHAPTER 30

Self-Determination

It's a long way from the bedroom to the kitchen
when all the thought in back of thought is loss.
How wide the dark rooms are you walk across
with a glass of water and a migraine
tablet. Sweat of hard dreams: unforgiven
silences, missed opportunities.
The night progresses like chronic disease,
symptom by symptom, sentences without pardon.
        —MARILYN HACKER, from "Migraine Sonnets"

Marilyn Hacker explores the ways in which depression replicates the condition and experience of having a migraine headache. She analogizes a night of suffering alone through a migraine to the psychological state of grief over the loss of a lover. Here, the mind does not control the body but rather shares experiences with it, as both the psychological and physical selves feel and sense pain the same way. Mental and visceral responses are, in Hacker's poem, akin, working in tandem.

Is it then such a surprise that I had experienced dysphoria, dysthymia, depression, anxiety, and solipsistic thinking in that first year? And, yet, one of the psychological diagnoses made at the clinic was that I was suffering from an "adjustment disorder with depressed mood." I had to look up that one; it seems that there is a "normal" way to respond to chronic pain and an "abnormal" way. Yours truly was apparently handling her chronic pain in a decidedly abnormal manner. I am grateful for Hacker's poem. It acted as a corrective, made me doubt this diagnosis, and stopped me from labeling my behavior as aberrant and thereby blaming myself. The poem further helped me to understand my psychological responses as forgivable, normal given the circumstances (even inevitable—who would have handled the year better, I self-defensively ask myself).

The psychological report also labeled me as having certain "personality traits and [a] coping style" that negatively impacted my head pain, namely "dependent" and "obsessive/compulsive" personality traits. The doctors had diagnosed me as having a dependent personality primarily on the account of one nurse who tried to teach me to self-inject Toradol, the anti-inflammatory medication, on my last day in the hospital. Rushing to make a flight home, I had explained to her that five of my sisters- and brothers-in-law were doctors and worked within two blocks of my house. I would never need to self-administer a shot. She apparently told my psychologist that I had refused to learn the procedure (leaving out this critical detail about my family), and so I suddenly had become a "dependent" personality, a personality type perversely dissident with my own perceived personality type as the "histrionic caretaker" of my family. These three personality types had all been discussed at the clinic in a class devoted to "Personality Patterns and Pain," as they apparently create special problems for the acute pain patient. Now, honestly, how can one person be all three of these types (as well as the fourth type, "narcissistic," which in my mind seemed to suit me even better)?

At my first follow-up visit back at the clinic two months after my discharge, I, in the words of my doctor, "obsessively/compulsively debated these psychological diagnoses." I finally broke him down enough to agree that one simply couldn't be all of these types at the same time. Conceding on the obsessive/compulsive trait, I later jabbed an anti-inflammatory shot into my leg in front of a nurse, thereby dispelling my categorization as "dependent."

Why was it so important to me to debate my mental diagnoses? Why did I care whether or not they thought I was off my rocker? Again, I think it got back to the same question that had absorbed me all fall—did my mental state somehow cause my physical state? I had always been high-strung, a cat on a hot tin roof. Yet I started thinking that it was all too simplistic, a knee-jerk reaction even, for a doctor to blame my pain loop on psychological problems. I admittedly have a type A, high-octane, overachieving personality, but I had never suffered from headaches before now. Further, there had been far more stressful periods in my life when I had had nary a headache. Of one thing I have become quite sure—this pain is physiological.

Acute pain sufferers routinely relate how doctors dismiss their pain as imaginary, unsolvable, or psychosomatically induced. Doctors, discouraged themselves by their inability to cure the pain, will too often take their irritation out on the patient. I looked back on the many doctors whom I had allowed to infiltrate my instincts and question my mental stability as having done damage. So I vowed that, going forward, I would no longer permit doctors to apply their own narratives to my story; I would script it for myself.

CHAPTER 31

Fissures

I struck the board, and cried, No more.
　　　　　I will abroad.
　What? shall I ever sigh and pine?
My lines and life are free; free as the road,
　Loose as the wind, as large as store. . . .

But as I raved and grew more fierce and wild
　　　　At every word,
Me thoughts I heard one calling, Childe:
　And I replied, My Lord.
—GEORGE HERBERT, from "The Collar"

One of the most satisfying attributes of seventeenth-century Protestant minds is how unself-consciously they admit to hesitations, uncertainties, even fissures in their faith. They describe in countless diaries, meditations, and confessional poems like Herbert's "The Collar" their ongoing, ever-present battles with doubt. These doubts are not prim or restrained but rather "fierce and wild." Their efforts to stay firm in their faith are willed exercises, conscious and forced struggles to dispel disbelief. Herbert even refers to God's hold on him as a "collar," with all of its attendant psychological associations—choler, strain, subordination, rebellion—and physical manifestations: the cleric's collar, a dog collar, a slave's manacles. The end of "The Collar" feels like resignation, stooping before God's stronger will, and a forced acceptance of the master-servant role, as much as it brings peace to the poet and closure to the poem. I, too, have found my optimism and faith in recovery shaky and inconstant. Uncertainty perhaps accompanies the process of healing for all of us. Will we get better? How much will we get better? What will we do if we don't get better? Hope proves slippery in such moments, wiggling out of hands, slipping through fingers. Hope refuses reification, comes and goes, turns solid, then liquid. It morphs from fire into water, from air into earth.

Doubt is hardest for me to expel in the wake of continuing problems. I realized recently that my personality has changed in the face of chronic pain, or, at least, that I make a different impression on people. I come off as a tad spacey and flitty. If I haven't lost my cell phone that day or left my purse in a restaurant, then I have forgotten about plans I have made. I also tend to avoid probing questions and, at times, choose superficiality when words evade me. I am too often still plagued by memory losses as well and continue to behave like Mrs. Malaprop, a character in Richard Sheridan's play *The Rivals*, who ridiculously misuses words. (My favorite line in the play is her comment "He is the very pineapple of politeness.") In the spring, I fluctuated between thinking that my malapropisms were due to my brian's lack of exercise during the past year or to the opioids still operating on my brain chemistry. Alternatively, I reasoned that my continued use of Klonopin accounted for my mental fuzziness. Prescribed by my neurologist to treat ongoing withdrawal symptoms, Klonopin is usually prescribed to treat anxiety disorders. One of its key side effects is "impaired coordination and memory."

Now, no longer going through withdrawal or taking Klonopin, I tend to attribute my continuing lack of mental acuity to another, more disturbing potential cause. The headache clinic recently conducted a study that demonstrates that head pain can cause memory and concentration problems. Barbaranne Branca, author of the article "Headaches and Memory," reports that headache pain patients experience "cognitive inefficiency, confusion, and problems with thinking clearly." Further, patients often have "[p]roblems with speech production, stuttering, word-finding problems, decreased vocabulary, completion of sentences, and mathematical computation."

Whatever the cause of my ongoing memory losses, they continue to affect my everyday functioning. I spent one afternoon walking up and down Central Park West looking for a doctor's office recently, because I had forgotten to bring the address with me. I didn't know how to spell the doctor's complicated last name (Deliyannides) and so couldn't call information. I was sure that I knew where her office was, yet it took eleven blocks of walking to find the building. Then I couldn't find my doctor's name on the bell. I did see another name on the buzzer that looked oddly familiar, although I wasn't sure that I recognized it. Only later would I realize that I had conflated two of my doctors' offices and had ended up at a hypnotist's office to whom I had gone (ineffectually) a few times earlier that month. It surprised me that I had neither remembered her name nor her office. Was it my medication's fault? The pain's fault? Maybe the hypnosis? The incident does serve in many ways as a leitmotif for me—symbolizing all of the other confusions, fruitless wanderings, and ill-conceived journeys of the past two years.

Worse, my cognitive lapses have led to embarrassing, if not painful, social encounters. With the advent of early summer, our little street bloomed. Families hidden inside in the winter months and rainy spring now began to emerge and reconnect. One such evening, I introduced two neighbors, bowdlerizing both of their names—John became Jack (actually his son's name); Fran Edson became simply Mrs. Edelman, as I had completely forgotten her first name (even though I have known her for more than a decade). The conversation that ensued with John led to my remembrance of a poem that I used to know by heart. "It's by Theodore Roethke," I said, trying to prod his memory as well as my own. I apparently mispronounced Roethke, and the man casually corrected me, also mentioning that he had known Roethke personally as a boy and that Roethke had even written a poem about him. What could be more embarrassing?! Now even more determined to jog my memory, I said, "I can't keep talking to you until I find that poem." I went into my house, grabbing the book in which I knew the poem appeared, and ran back outside to show it to him. To my chagrin, I found that the poem was not by Roethke, but rather by Dylan Thomas. I had conflated two distinctly different poems, "The Waking" by Theodore Roethke and "Do Not Go Gentle into That Good Night" by Dylan Thomas. They shared neither thematic subject matter nor philosophy. The poems had only one attribute in common: they were both villanelles.

These sorts of addled bunglings, while at times forgivable, even amusing in the absurdity of their entanglements, at other times smacked of sheer inconsiderateness. The occasion that still makes me cringe most also involved a neighbor. I saw her rushing down the sidewalk one evening looking quite distressed. When I asked her if there was anything wrong, and if I could help, she replied, obviously quite upset, "Mike just got into a car accident and is at the hospital." I looked at her blankly. "Who is Mike?" I asked. "My husband," she nearly shrieked and kept running. Of course, I knew his name. It had, at that moment, however, completely evaporated. Finding me so unforgivably lame, she called upon other neighbors and friends that night to help her, and for that, I feel both remorseful and helpless. So much for helping someone else for a change.

My memory losses, as they continue in both small and large ways, often attack my defensive efforts to remain stalwart and positive. Creeping into my mind camouflaged, the doubts ambush me. I had actually thought before my gaffe with my neighbor that I was having an interesting conversation about poetry with him, relieved finally to be discussing my favorite topic again, only to feel deflated, even humiliated, afterward. My former ease with and grasp of poetry had fled. These mental agitations led to even larger doubts. How would I be able to return to teaching? How would I be able to remember the names of ninety students each semester? How would I be able to draw upon my reserves of poetry, as I had so often in the past, casually reciting a line or stanza of a poem in class when the conversation had spontaneously led to the perfect quotation? This technique, I knew, excited students, emphasizing for them the wealth of insights one could find in poetry and the importance—the necessity even—of having poetry in their lives. How, if I couldn't even remember the poems themselves, would I be able to lead a class discussion?

This "dysfunctional" thinking, as the clinic's therapist would undoubtedly have exclaimed had she heard this inner monologue, I find unavoidable. While I know never to reside in that space permanently anymore, I still return there for mini visits. I open the door, peek inside, feel the cold blast, and then know to shut the door again. I have, apparently, more Puritan leanings than I had originally thought.

CHAPTER 32

Acceptance

I wake to sleep, and take my waking slow.
I feel my fate in what I cannot fear.
I learn by going where I have to go.

We think by feeling. What is there to know?
I hear my being dance from ear to ear.
I wake to sleep, and take my waking slow.

Of those so close beside me, which are you?
God bless the Ground! I shall walk softly there,
And learn by going where I have to go.

Light takes the Tree; but who can tell us how?
The lowly worm climbs up a winding stair;
I wake to sleep, and take my waking slow.

Great Nature has another thing to do
To you and me, so take the lively air,
And, lovely, learn by going where to go.

This shaking keeps me steady. I should know.
What falls away is always. And is near.
I wake to sleep, and take my waking slow.
I learn by going where I have to go.
    —THEODORE ROETHKE, "The Waking"

Perhaps it was propitious that I had conflated Roethke's and Dylan Thomas's villanelles in my conversation with my neighbor. Roethke's "The Waking" has become a defining palindrome, offering me, paradoxically, both clarity and unanswerable questions. This response is appropriate somehow, as Roethke structures the poem on paradoxes.

At my two-month follow-up visit at the headache clinic, my neurologists remained upbeat, and we spent a great deal of time mapping out changes to my medications that could address my continuingly high pain levels. They were particularly heartened by my improved mental state and functionality. They also cautioned that this was a process of "baby steps," of trying new medications slowly and creatively playing with them in terms of dosages and timing. This process could take several months before we found the right combination of both preventative and abortive medications. They also cautioned that this process did not have a sure outcome—whether I would get 40 percent or 80 percent better, it was still impossible to say. They, nevertheless, had great hopes for me and promised to devote themselves to my continuing care.

My appointment with the pain anesthesiologist the next day did not go as well. He discussed with me the results of my two RF ablation procedures. He divulged what I hadn't known until then—that my fusion surgeon had indeed made burning the C2 nerve extremely difficult. He said that he had studied the nerves on both sides with fluoroscopic guidance but had found so much hardware in my neck and wires wrapped so tightly together, that he could not access the nerve from either side. The nerve was simply buried in the fusion. This had been my fear for months— at times assuaged, at times forgotten—that I would now have intractable nerve pain, because the nerves were perhaps permanently damaged and inaccessible. Here, finally, had been a doctor who had gone in and aggressively tried to get at the nerve. To no avail.

Confirmation of my situation would prove as relentlessly opaque as all prior attempts at diagnoses. My neurosurgeon definitively denied that the C2 nerve could be causing pain since the surgery. My anesthesiologist in New York disagreed and further thought that it was worth trying to access the nerve again— a different machine, different technique, different angles, different doctor. This information, nevertheless, had a profound impact on me. It ended an era, announced a finality that until now had been evaded or put off. One could no longer say with certainty that my condition had a surefire cure. No longer could I continue looking for the next doctor, the next procedure, the next drug to cure me. There would be no one medical procedure that could single-handedly alleviate all of my symptoms and make me whole again.

So I found myself in a new place. It was one of acceptance, a giving in, a letting go, accompanied by a firm faith in endurance. The project now was to accept that "what falls away is always." I could no longer stand the constant focus on getting better. The I of yesterday is not the I of now. My self had changed, and I had to learn to live with myself and with this change. So, too, this body was uncharted, unfamiliar. I didn't belong in it, and it didn't belong to me. Yet I had waited actively for my body to return to its former health, and it hadn't. I did not recognize, understand, or like this new body; nevertheless, I had to own it, to make it mine. I might not be able to dance as I had, but I could still "hear my being dance from ear to ear." I would "walk softly," finally changing courses. The epic quest needed to end or, at least, I needed to embark on a new quest. I have a condition that is chronic; "what [else] is there to know?" I could no longer deny it, berate it, grieve it, flee from it, be terrorized by it, fight it.

Instead of focusing on a cure, I would place my energy into healing—in all of its varied forms. I would practice calm. I would search for inner resolve. My body and soul had been unmade—it was now time to remake myself and put back together those parts of myself that felt fragmented, split, and broken at the core. I indeed did "wake to sleep" and would find this condition tenable only by easing into it. I would need to continue re-educating myself, changing directions, and recovering slowly. My unmaking had been sudden and unforeseen. Why it had occurred remained an enigma. The process of remaking would be slow and tedious. It was the best that I could do in the face of a changed life—one that I didn't want, hadn't asked for, but now must finally learn to manage.

"And must I then, indeed, Pain, live with you / All through

my life?—sharing my fire, my bed, / Sharing—oh, worst of all things!—the same head?— / . . . So be it, then, if what seems true is true: / Let us to dinner, comrade, and be fed" (Edna St. Vincent Millay, "clxxiv"). Millay's poem beautifully captures an aspect of acceptance that has been critical to me: the resolution to continue to live through and with the pain. The poem demonstrates so many of the ways in which pain can invade the psyche. I relate to the speaker describing pain as living with her, as I too feel that pain is always present—I can't shake it. Somehow in this poem, though, the speaker manages to overcome pain's omnipresent hovering and refuses to allow pain to continue behaving, in my friend Jillisa's words, like some kind of parasitic, pillaging squatter, taking her hearth, home, and even her bed. She resolves instead to be hospitable and comes to invite Pain to her table. The poem models not simply resignation, but true equability. In the presence of pain, one somehow curtsies and learns to waltz with it.

I observed firsthand how one could choose not mere submission but open acceptance at the New York City Ballet in the early summer. The evening was a milestone moment—a formal farewell to and final performance of Kyra Nichols, the prima ballerina whose career at NYCB spanned over thirty years. NYCB's tradition allows the retiring dancer to choose the program for the evening. Her final choice I consider one of the great moments in Balanchine's choreography, that portion of *Vienna Waltzes* when the stage, set to replicate a grand ballroom, fills with waltzing dancers. The men in black tuxedos, the women in white satin ball gowns, diamond necklaces, and long white gloves. As they waltz, the women lift the trains of their dresses to create fans of swirling, twirling satin, and the speed of the waltz transforms them into whirling dervishes of joy.

The piece ended. The audience jumped to its feet applauding and roaring "Brava!" Tiny Kyra Nichols stepped forward alone to the center of the stage, beaming, and curtsied low. The entire company joined in the applause for her, and I found it particularly moving to see her fellow dancers publicly honor her. Then one man after another—the director of the company, her son, her partners—presented her with enormous bouquets of roses. She hugged each man, set the bouquet down on the floor, only in time for the next man to present her with another bouquet. The audience began flinging bouquets onto the stage as well, and then the heavens opened, and rose petals, pink glitter, and confetti wafted onto the stage all around her. What I had anticipated would be an evening of bittersweet good-byes and tears became an evening of joyous acceptance and roses. Flowers blooming, hope growing, promises still waiting to be fulfilled. This moment continues to have a powerful effect on me. I had the same option and choice before me as Nichols. If this great ballerina could so gracefully say good-bye to her old life, then I could learn to do so as well. I might have chosen mere resignation, but in the interests of goodwill, of free will, of good coming of my will, I willed myself to choose acceptance instead.

CHAPTER 33

Parties, Drugs, and Rock and Roll

I can't get no satisfaction.
—THE ROLLING STONES, from "Satisfaction"

Puritan in thinking at times, I nevertheless devolved into the anathema of a good Puritan that spring—for one night, at Holly's book party, I became a party girl. A real New York party, replete with top-tier socialites, novelists, publishers, PR divas, gossip columnists, news anchors, and billionaires, it celebrated the publication of Holly's first novel.

Somehow in the girls-gone-wild atmosphere of the party, a group of us began talking about drugs—mother's little helpers, antidepressants, and then the illicit. Unexpectedly, one of the women mentioned that she had some pot with her. Marijuana was the one drug for pain relief that I had not tried, and it had been making headlines that spring. Connecticut had introduced a bill legalizing its use for medicinal purposes. Not yet state law, the bill had generated a significant amount of media attention and been publicly both vilified and strongly supported. To relieve pain in cancer patients, doctors had long prescribed Marinol, a pill meant to emulate synthetically the main chemical in marijuana. Even Marinol is considered controversial, and most states have fairly rigid licensing laws controlling its usage. I had not thought much of Marinol as an option, nor had a doctor suggested it to me. All I knew about it was that most studies concluded that pot was the more effective analgesic.

Until that evening, only two people had suggested pot to me. Both were parents of friends of mine, well into their sixties and by all standards conservative. I guess I should have assumed that anyone who attended college in the sixties must have known something about drugs, gray flannel suits and sensible heels notwithstanding. They had both thought that I should at least try pot to see if it dulled my pain in the same way that it worked for cancer patients. I had found their suggestions amusing but had never taken them seriously; I, it turned out, more conservative than they.

That night, however, I decided to take their advice, primarily because my friend offered to share her pot with me. Like teenagers, we spent a fruitless period searching for a place to smoke it, laughing as we flew about the party trying to behave surreptitiously. We ended up outside of the restaurant, huddled under an awning in the rain, but we weren't alone. Paparazzi from an online blog had descended to photograph the evening. Oblivious to the photographers, still assuming that I was a Nobody, I couldn't understand why my friend kept telling me to turn around and act cool while we smoked. I drew a particularly deep breath, overly fascinated at the white paper melting to gray torch, and passed the joint back to her. Fascinated neither by the joint nor by my behavior, she seemed annoyed and went back inside. No matter, I thought, as I proceeded to finish the entire joint myself. The shot of me busily smoking the vestiges of the joint, holding the roach with my pinkie outstretched in my designer dress, did make the Web site's headlines the next day. Another snapshot of the year.

Always excessive in this period when it came to drugs, I behaved no differently that evening. I had forgotten how much one should smoke and had smoked far, far too much. It might as well have been three hundred ninety-two clicks on the morphine pump. And stoned I was. Billie Holiday stoned. Grateful Dead stoned. So stoned, in fact, that I had a brief revelatory epiphany, à la Jim Morrison in the desert. I thought that I was pain free. I couldn't feel anything, except a nice buzzing and tingling in my nerve endings.

"It's a miracle," I kept repeating, floating about the party as, for the first time in nearly a year, I didn't have a headache. Eric and brother-in-law Nick, amused but also worried that I would fall into a plant, walked around with me as I kept muttering, "It's a miracle." Jeanne was so thrilled by this news that I thought she would start crying. Instead, she got out her cell phone and scored my next stash. She ran out of the party to fetch it during dinner, and I arrived home with a nice little bag of weed tucked into my satin evening purse.

At the party, my state of euphoria lasted for about forty-five minutes. While it worked exceptionally well to rid me of pain during that period, what I had not anticipated was how it also managed to swell and intensify my emotions—not just for forty-five minutes, but for several hours. After losing the husbands, I found myself reefer-madnessing all over the respectable wood-paneled restaurant, horrifying anyone who dared engage me. Throughout the evening, friends and acquaintances approached me, wanting to hear how I was faring. Party-girl rules be damned, if they asked how I was doing, they got the truth. I would launch into a dramatic rant about how it was unbearable to live in such pain, and, by the way, I had also given up expecting any kind of cure. Confused expressions gave way to forced smiles. "No," they would respond trying to muster sincerity, "in every great human story, before there is eternal hope, there is lost hope." They thought that they were just witnessing a particularly grief-stricken stage along a continuing trajectory. Somehow, they assured themselves, I would rise to the occasion and find a cure for my pain. My black hole, sucking in so many well-meaning friends and acquaintances, continued throughout the evening, until finally it gave way to a full-blown tragi-fest at dinner with my best friends—gulpy sobs, runny nose, head on the table.

The next morning, feeling awful physically, I chiefly felt embarrassed by my conduct at the party. Within hours of awakening, my phone went berserk with calls from various family members who, hearing that the pot had taken away my pain, were ecstatic that I had finally found an efficacious painkiller. My mother announced that she had no problem with one of her daughters becoming a pothead. Who cared whether I was a little bit melodramatic, if I was feeling no pain? A couple of friends called to say that they could get more pot for me. Jeanne, who admitted that I had smoked way too much, wanted me to begin smoking pot with clinical precision. I should conduct a scientific experiment. First, try smoking only one puff and see if that was enough to dull the pain. If not, then I should continue trying, adding only one puff at a time incrementally to determine the correct "dosage."

Nothing could have been more absurd from my perspective. The pot had left me as loopy as any of the other medications I had tried that year. Another night of having lost my brain. I was still, perhaps, lucid enough to carry on conversations with people, but I had behaved with absolutely no control. It had brought out my depressed side—even my paranoid side. Again, I was dealing with side effects and found them simply intolerable given my shaky psychological state.

Insistent that many doctors considered pot one of the most reliable painkillers around, Jeanne refused to surrender. She coerced our friend, a cook who particularly loves baking, to experiment with how to cook pot into food. He first tried cookies but opted ultimately for the old-fashioned pot brownie, perfecting a recipe that he hoped would create a subtler, less intense high than smoking. He came over carrying a plate stacked with them. We had a pot brownie dinner party with friends who agreed to participate in our experiment that same night. One brownie . . . nothing. Two brownies . . . nothing. Three brownies . . . a slight buzziness but mostly an enormous stomachache from having eaten so much. Too subtle a high, pot again proved a failure.

I experimented with pot a third and final time with my sister Jeanne. This time, we decided to try the scientific approach initially suggested by her. Hiding in my garden, we huddled together over our stash. When we first opened the package, the dried leaves misled us; they didn't look or smell like our memory of pot. Perhaps, we thought, they were the latest or some rare and particularly exotic variety. We began pulling out the dried leaves and stacking them on top of a thin sheet of rolling paper—only to discover on closer inspection that what we were rolling was pot-pourri. The real pot had been expertly camouflaged, hidden in a small bag at the center of the innocent dried leaves. We were equally inept at rolling the joint, if that is the correct word for the lopsided and lumpy-looking sausage that required our combined efforts to mold. We forged ahead and methodically tried one puff at a time synchronized by long pauses in between in order to calibrate the exact pitch of our high. Once I had attained a perfect balance—no pain, but not too stoned—we would stop.

Or so we had planned. Until we heard sobbing, and Lilly came flying out into the garden. She was shrieking at me, "Smoking?! You are smoking?! You are going to die!" High-pitched wails of "Stooooooooop" and more hysteria. Of course, we immediately put it out and then tried to explain to her that I was not smoking a cigarette but rather "an herb" that could help with my pain. She was beyond reason and inconsolable for the rest of the afternoon. Nothing soothed her. Nothing pacified her rage and fear. She was adamant that I swear never, ever to smoke again. (At least, I admit, I have filed this argument away to drag out when she's a teenager and I might need to use it against her.) My usually sweet daughter said that she didn't care if it might make me feel better. My family was surprised by her lack of compassion; I tried to understand her reaction as an indicator of how she had internalized my injury. Did she really worry that I would die? When I tried to talk about what had happened in a calmer moment, she refused to elaborate. Her explosive emotions were beyond her ability either to control or to discuss. In my mind, this event marked another shift in Lilly, another tearing of the soul.

Needless to say, I vowed never to smoke pot again and made a big show of throwing away the bag of weed. The risks of further damaging Lilly far outweighed the palliative benefits of continuing to smoke. This reality check sent my family into a tailspin, as I firmly announced that pot was yet another magical elixir that, like so many of the others, indeed burned but also crashed.

CHAPTER 34

Fallout

"Nothing lasts"—
how bitterly the thought attends each loss.

"Nothing lasts"—
a promise also of consolation

Grief and hope
the skipping rope's two ends,
twin daughters of impatience.

One wears a dress of wool, the other cotton.
—JANE HIRSHFIELD, "Nothing Lasts"

How to make a person feel safe and stable? Wasn't it Eric's and my responsibility to provide such security for our children? I worried that since the beginning of this ordeal, Benjamin and Lilly had learned only the harsh lesson that "nothing lasts" but grief, and that I had failed to offer the "promise also of consolation." I remembered few occasions the whole first year in which we had skipped rope for hope, joy, or even just fun. The first year our family faced what my friend Paula describes as "triage"; the intensity simply of surviving took over all else. Fallout describes the second year.

The bickering between brother and sister that had developed in the first year continued into the second; their behavior toward Eric and me, however, began to shift. The tactics of the two kids differed. Benjamin tended toward diplomacy and peacemaking. He tried to pacify whoever was upset. When anger turned in his direction, he would fold immediately and mildly apologize— sometimes for nothing—in order to smooth out our anger. Becoming a teenager already marked such a defining moment in his life. Had our year of crisis changed him irrevocably from the man he would have become? Would he now play peacemaker in all of his significant relationships—particularly with women? He punctuated sentences with a hopeful "I love you" so often that it became almost an involuntary hiccup. I would respond, "You're a charmer," and he would grin that goofy, nearing handsome smile. Other times he melded like wallpaper into the background. For such a naturally rambunctious kid, to withdraw so completely must have taken a tremendous act of self-control, and he must have felt under terrible compulsion to do so.

Lilly's behavior and moods continued to morph. We noticed a new shift one evening when Eric was trying to give me a shot of Toradol in the bathroom. I had become so needle phobic that I could no longer inject myself. Making a fuss about even Eric giving me the shot, I was shrieking a bit and jumping out of his way every time he tried to push the needle in. "Damn it!" I yelped when Eric finally stabbed me successfully. Just then, from down the hall, we heard Lilly shouting, "Don't yell at Daddy! Leave him alone!" She was in a state. Convinced that we were having an argument, she instinctively blamed me. I explained to her that I needed the shots to control the pain, but that I didn't like getting shots any more than she did. I also explained that I hadn't been angry at Daddy—just having a difficult time getting the shot. "I'm sorry that I got you worried." Suddenly, she burst into tears and threw herself on top of me. I didn't know why. Did she feel guilty? Scared? Empathic? All I could whisper to her over and over again was "I'm sorry, Lilly goat. I'm so, so sorry."

Overwhelmed by the intensity and constant fluctuation of her emotions, I found myself unable to steady her in this period. My only recourse was to rely on inadequate apologies. The most extreme instance took place at Benjamin's bar mitzvah. During the service, the rabbi led the congregation in the Prayer for Healing. This prayer came as a surprise to me as did the manner of reciting it; I could not remember ever having heard it before. The rabbi invited individual members of the congregation to step forward and speak out loud the name of the person to whom one wanted to dedicate the prayer. Again and again, I heard my name, whispered by family members, proclaimed by Jewish and non-Jewish friends alike. In the middle of this litany, Lilly lunged at me, weeping. Her face buried in my chest, I found myself again repeating the inadequate mantra, "I'm sorry, Lilly. I'm so, so sorry." I had been good at comforting her in the past; I had always been the person to whom she turned when upset, tired, or scared. She still turned to me in those vulnerable moments, but I could not always provide the solace I had in the past. I was so often the cause of her distress in the first place.

This stage—bereavement, perhaps—lasted only a season. By fall in the second year of my pain, tears had given way to anger. Her life had changed, perhaps irrevocably, without her consent, and she didn't like it. "Why are you wearing that neck collar? You don't need to anymore. Take it off." "Why are you not better yet?" "You're always talking about your neck." Eric observed that I too often sank to her level, altogether abdicating my parental authority. I had lost my empathy and seemed only to escalate the rows. Underneath both of our anger, I knew, lurked fear, hurt, loss. Her grief was so raw and daily exacerbated by my continuing and noticeable problems that I knew she needed to establish some independence from me. I was no longer as accessible; she needed a more reliable source of parental support and so began to turn to her father. I, too, needed some separation, as I instinctively knew that I couldn't always give her what she wanted anymore; yet this was too painful a realization, and I preferred to bury it under anger.

My moods also fluctuated with my pain. On some spike days, proper mothering simply couldn't happen. I continued to seal myself off from her. Sometimes she rebelled against this tendency and would insist upon being with me anyway. Our engagements in these moments were fraught. She insisted on chattering with me, but, so phonosensitive, I sometimes found the conversation difficult to tolerate and would get irritated, cut her off, lose my temper. On better days, I could be lavish in my nurturing, trying to make up for the difficult days and enclose her in a womb of security. These mood swings, not clearly understood by her as pain driven, left her stable core teetering.

That fall, I also employed a range of daily strategies to cope with her anger, too often flipping between extreme reactions, thereby perpetuating my unreliability. Sometimes I would cave. "I understand that you are upset with me, Lilly. This must be so hard for you." Sometimes, I would refuse to engage. "I am going to leave this room before either of us says something that we will regret." More often, I found it impossible not to lose my temper. "You may *not* talk that way to me; I am your mother!" How awful, this truism. It didn't reflect on my level of maturity or control or on my ability to rise above the fray. All it confirmed was that I would always win our fights, simply because I was bigger than she and so could yell louder.

I'm not sure why I had so little tolerance. Perhaps I felt sensitive, too, and got my feelings hurt, as I interpreted her anger as a lack of compassion toward me. Perhaps because, growing up, we received harsh rebukes from my father for any disrespect shown to our mother. It rankled me that I did not garner the same respect as had my mother. Or perhaps because our own family dynamic had positioned me as the bad cop to Eric's good cop. Instinct turned into habit. I naturally wanted to reprimand; Eric wanted to placate. There was nobody to establish limits to Lilly's behavior, except for me, which only made her angrier.

My uncle Sandy and cousin Lilly came over one evening for a drink. Chattering in the living room, we were talking about all of the good restaurants that had opened in Brooklyn. My uncle made a joke about how this would be good for me, as I so rarely cooked. Lilly piped in, teasing me about my bad cooking as well. I became incensed, hearing that edge of aggression I had heard far too often of late, and yelled at her in front of everyone for her lack of respect. She shut down and didn't talk the rest of the evening. I had struck another blow.

Another evening, my parents came over for dinner; long after we had eaten and close to Lilly's bedtime, Eric walked in from work. My parents and I had known that he would not make it home in time for dinner, as he had a work commitment that evening. When he walked in, Lilly sidled up to me and whispered, "Well, that was really mean, Mom, not to wait for Daddy to eat. Now he has to eat alone, by himself." My mother, overhearing her, got upset this time. "I think it's mean for you to talk that way to your mother—and mean of you to expect that your grandparents should have to wait until nine-thirty at night to eat dinner, Lilly. You owe your mother an apology." The blowout, as per usual, escalated. Lilly, raging, then crying, then simply done in, fell asleep upstairs in the middle of her time-out. We had traded empathy for a no-tolerance rigidity, an approach that didn't seem to do anybody any good.

We had lost our foundation. The architecture of our family dynamic, seismically shifting and wobbling all year, now finally collapsed. The anger had taken us both hostage and by surprise. How to purge ourselves of it? I realized how easy it is to do damage, to cause ruin. Slide just that little bit off the cliff, and it would prove impossible to climb back to a level of stability. To her credit, my daughter had held it together for over a year, enduring months of distressing events any one of which alone could traumatize a child—my unhappiness and unavailability, the hideous trip to Florida, the dog dying, my extended hospital stay, the difficult visit, and my returning home after all of that so little improved. Why did her crisis begin, though, just when I was making so much of an effort to be available and functional again? Perhaps her delayed response indicates how mentally healthy she had formerly been. Or perhaps the delay indicates that she thought it was finally safe to show her anger, because I no longer seemed as precarious.

I had spent the first year so sick that I had been unable to focus on anything outside of my ravaged body and so had tattered the intricate weave of familial relations, that fragile web that bound our family together. I began to see that this self-involvement, while perhaps unavoidable at first, was not just inconsiderate, but dishonorable. Those children needed me to deal and to do so with compassion.

This was the first time in thirteen years of parenting that I found myself unequipped to handle a situation. I had neither the skills and training nor the stamina to repair these rips alone. The only option seemed to be to turn to outside counseling to navigate the intense shifts and emotions that gripped our family.

While we may never regain our old family dynamic, we are currently working hard to attain a more stable one. We have more hindsight than we had before, more coping skills. Mostly, we have a deep longing to reconnect with one another. Sometimes I think that my children, although stained, have also grown from this crisis. They have learned independence, compassion, and a lesson in life's sometimes difficult realities. Eric and I do believe that they both know how much we love them. For now, though, our family remains a house under construction; the relationships at times rise to a level of harmony and affectionate ease, and at other times are still fractured, still fractious.

CHAPTER 35

The Fall into Life

We try a new drug, a new combination
of drugs, and suddenly
I fall into my life again. . . .
    —JANE KENYON, from "Back"

꧁꧂ Although I have ostensibly given up hope of finding a cure for my condition, I still continue to explore new treatment options. Throughout the second year a.p., my pain anesthesiologist tried different shots to reduce my pain—facet nerve blocks at C3, C4, C5, and occipital nerves again as well as cervical plexus blocks. He also decided at least to try the RF ablation at C2, even though the other pain doctor had not been able to access it.

With nothing to lose, but little expectation, I underwent the block fairly indifferently. Rigorously laid-back, impervious to the procedure, I didn't even have Eric stay with me to hold my hand, take me home, or get me settled in bed. I simply had him come at the end of the procedure to help me get into a cab. He went back to work, and I went home by myself.

At the end of the procedure, the doctor triumphantly announced that, while difficult to get close to the nerve on the left side because of all the wiring, he had come perhaps close enough to it to have some effect. Even better, he had definitely gotten in on the right side. With this news, for all of my efforts to remain apathetic, I found myself just that little bit positive. I waited for two weeks—and then the not-even-dared-to-be-hoped-for result sneaked in, creeping up on me a little every day . . .

Ten days. Ten inexpressibly beautiful days. I have no words for that caesura. Only a poet like Jane Kenyon could describe this ineffable "fall into my life again." Normalcy—impossibly precious normalcy. The taste of pure, cold water. Simple clearheadedness and a kind of buoyancy. I no longer felt an iron weight on my head.

I did everything in my power to prolong this nonfeeling. I didn't travel—by plane, car, or on foot. I did no exercise, no physical therapy. I got no massages and tried not to move my neck. I lay low, continued my naps, and didn't strain myself. I tiptoed through my days.

So fragile, this hush of nonpain. Useless to dwell on desire cut short. The pain came back, worse than ever. A constant spike for eight days, the longest one I had yet experienced. Why, I am not sure. The doctor, nevertheless encouraged by the ten-day respite, repeated the injection. Another ascent of hope and another vacation from pain—twelve days this time—but then its return. A giant crush to the skull. I went down again.

My doctor, luckily quite gifted at wielding a needle, remains optimistic. He and my neurologist definitely think that I am experiencing neuropathic pain. In their opinion, my C1 and/or C2 nerves were somehow stretched or damaged. Whether such damage is permanent or not, it is impossible to say, and even if the injury has already healed, the nerve continues to send pain signals to the brain, thereby perpetuating the cycle of pain. While such pain is notoriously difficult to treat, my pain anesthesiologist refuses to give up.

We all recognize at this point that no one shot, procedure, drug, or operation will single-handedly take away the pain permanently; nevertheless, there exist options that can help manage the pain for finite periods. After something like forty ineffectual nerve and joint injections (I have honestly lost count of the exact number), I am now "on the margins" of treatment options. Most of the options left are exponentially more invasive and, in some cases, painful, so I continue to "take my waking slow." I schedule subsequent procedures when I have the muscle to go through with them. Other options seem too experimental still, and I will not undergo them until the technology improves.

Tempering expectation, managing this middle position between acceptance of the permanent nature of this condition and continuing to work to bring the pain levels down, has required new psychological skills. In the summer, I turned for a period to meditation to provide the psychological support to handle this middle way. In order to learn more about meditation and how to do it, I initially took a series of introductory group classes from famed guru Sharon Salzberg. Her interpolation of meditation exercises with the rudiments of Buddhism was particularly helpful to me. The Buddhist concept of equanimity offered me yet another helpful principle by emphasizing that it is a mistake to find ourselves too invested in things beyond our control. Everything changes; nothing is reified or static. To accept this reality is to learn how to live with more harmony and not give in to feelings of desolation about those aspects of life beyond our personal influence. If pleasure/pain is one of the "eight primary vicissitudes of life," in Salzberg's words, then learning to accept this reality can lead to greater peace—of mind, of body, of soul. By my simply shifting my own perspective, looking through my mental telescope from a different angle, I can come to terms with my pain as simply that—pain. This view neutralizes the word, strips it of its associations with suffering, misery, hopelessness, at least at times. While pain is my reality, my mind can choose to see it in a myriad of ways.

This insight continues to resonate in my life, but I also find it somewhat incomplete. In some ways, this philosophy makes my present more bearable: if I can just change what I believe, convert, so to speak, then, I reason, I will be able to abide my reality. I, therefore, eagerly embrace this never-before-aspired-to philosophy. Another part of me, however, remains staunch, impervious, observing such grasping after newfangled principles as somewhat desperate. If one has never been a Buddhist, or even interested in Buddhism, then the striving toward it, in my case in midlife, feels somehow like a search after straws.

What I long for is to retain the essence of who I have always been. In Stanley Kunitz's words, "I have walked through many lives, / some of them my own, / and I am not who I was, / though some principle of being / abides . . ." ("The Layers"). Without that "principle of being," that sense of self, I feel lost. This process of "doing pain" has forced so much soul-searching, analysis, hard confrontations of myself, my behavior, my greatest fears, sorrows, and joys. Perhaps I am in the middle of a reframing, a reinvention, a rebirth; but, somehow, I think not. I think I am in the middle of just trying to keep myself in my life—flawed but, in essence, intact and still me.

Epilogue

CHAPTER 36

Rising

What makes the engine go?
Desire, desire, desire.
The longing for the dance
stirs in the buried life.
　　—STANLEY KUNITZ, from "Touch Me"

⟡ In November 2007, one year and five months after my life changed, I got out of bed. Such a simple act in so many ways, so ordinary, it required just a little shift of my thinking the morning it happened. I think I'll take Lil to school today and have coffee at Starbucks with my friends, I thought. In other ways, of course, it was a momentous shift.

My discharge papers from the hospital had included an instruction that I should spend twenty minutes a day performing an aerobic activity. Yet it took me six months after my discharge even to get out of bed. One of the side effects of having spent so long supine was that I had lost a great deal of overall strength; my muscles had atrophied to the point where I became fatigued just walking around the block. I began slowly—at first, the walk to Lilly's school and back was as far as I could go. I then ventured farther—the bank, the dry cleaner, the grocery store—and farther afield, ten blocks down the street, then twenty, then thirty. A mile became two miles. I started to make daily treks on the Brooklyn Bridge, at first only to its center, then all the way across and back.

The return of mobility catapulted me back into the world of the living, and I began slowly to regain my stamina. I found myself incrementally more functional over the course of several weeks and realized that the more time I spent out of bed, the more endurance and energy I had to stay out of it. By Christmas, I was strong enough to accompany my family on vacation. Before the trip, I had still felt feeble. Somehow, in that week, the sun and beach working their particular magic, I began to spend most of the day out of bed, needing only a late afternoon nap to regroup before getting up again to join everyone for dinner.

On one of the last days of the trip, I walked two miles in the heat with my iPod blasting the Rolling Stones and realized as I neared the end of the walk that I felt completely normal, that is, that I felt like myself before the pain—unself-consciously in my body, almost unaware, even, of my body. I had been lost in my thoughts and the music and the scenery for nearly an hour without having been pulled into my body and its problems. It was a kind of escapism and relief I had rarely experienced since the onset of pain.

As my strength returned, I found myself absorbed by the question of how I could replicate the experience of that walk—how to "taste the sweetness / of life in the center of pain" (Adrienne Rich, "New York"). Together, my sister Jackie and I determined that, as a priority, I needed to access endorphins regularly. There is a scientific rationale for seeking out endorphins, as they combat the brain chemistry that is reproducing pain signals. Flooding the brain with endorphins can thereby reduce pain. And, for those of us battling emotional issues as well as physical, an endorphin rush can relax a person faster than any antianxiety medication I have ever tried.

After a certain amount of trial and error, I determined that, at times, exercise and intense exertion give me access (at least I think) to endorphins. They somehow, if nothing else, distract me from feeling pain. It isn't that the pain goes away; it is still there, but it has receded into the background. I continue to walk, often three miles a day, but more meaningfully for me, I have also started dancing again. I used to sit outside the door of Benjamin's dance classes watching him as "longing for the dance" stirred in my "buried life." Emotional, moved by his grace, I equally lamented my own inability to take a ballet class anymore.

Pathos is no longer my approach. On most days I take a ballet class, usually a beginner class. Who cares what the level? I can't turn or do jumps anymore anyway. The beginner classes also have an advantage. Most of the class takes place at the barre rather than on the floor learning choreography. The barre work's attention to ballet technique allows me to concentrate fully on my form, strength, and flexibility. I also had a barre and full-length mirror put up in a small room that we previously used as storage space. I now go there on days when I don't have time for class. While I will never again move like a real dancer, my muscles have regained their prior mass and elasticity. My body no longer looks spindly but actually healthy and muscular, and Lilly has begun to tease me again about how I walk like a duck. Mostly, ballet, just as it did all of those years ago after my car accident, reminds me that I have a body that loves to move, reconnects me to grace (in all its meanings), and endows me with the capacity once again to feel grace-ful, grate-ful, full.

I also have a theory that ballet, by strengthening my spine and improving my posture, will help (and perhaps already helps) on some subtle level to realign my neck. Talking to other pain patients from the hospital, including men, I have found it interesting that many have turned to similar forms of exercise—especially yoga, Pilates, and stretch classes—since leaving the hospital. I don't think that this is accidental or a coincidence; rather, I think we have all unconsciously realized that these forms of exercise strengthen our cores and may even relieve pressure on whatever nerves are sending out distress signals.

By thinking about how my body was still capable of changing—this time, for the better—I also reconsidered physical therapy. It had been a fiasco after the surgery, primarily because I had been in too much pain and too drugged out to put any effort into it. With a certain amount of trepidation and not much expectation, I recommitted myself to physical therapy for several months. By going once a week, even though the surgery had taken place more than a year before, I managed to increase the mobility in my neck a little bit (not much, I admit, but definitely some). At least I no longer look like a robot or have to walk down the stairs sideways.

Endorphins are not my only means of finding physical pleasure again. I regularly get massages from Serena, who is also trained in meditation and a practicing Buddhist. I consider her a true healer. She will often talk me through relaxation exercises or meditations as she works on my neck. Sometimes she performs reflexology on my feet or Swedish massage on my back to address the muscle spasms induced by my rigid posture. Other days she massages my head and face to relieve my headaches or works on my neck aggressively, targeting pressure points to combat my nerve pain (oftentimes in the same places the acupuncturist had pricked me). No needles anymore—just cocoa butter, soothing music, and her kind hands.

A few more physical pleasures on which I rely are controversial: hot showers and cold compresses. Such simple measures, but for me they have worked. Some doctors caution that hot showers can spike head and neck pain. One should trust only cool showers. But where lies the joy in that? A steaming hot shower is a physical pleasure that I refuse to give up. Cold compresses, ice packs, freezing wet washcloths on my forehead, also feel delicious. Again, others swear by hot compresses and heating pads.

One of the other great luxuries in life, too often taken for granted, is sleep. I had never had a problem with sleep before, but pain initially turned me into an insomniac. Narcotics alleviated this problem, yet I had paid for their help with the side effect that the pills reversed my sleep patterns: awake all night, asleep all day. A permanent form of jet lag. At the time, I didn't want to "wake to sleep" and so was relieved that I could sleep the day away. Once off the pills, I found that I could still not sleep through the night. I usually awoke between 4:30 and 5:00 a.m., probably due to the pain at first, but it soon became my regular body clock. I would then need a nap by midafternoon.

At the clinic, the doctors had cautioned that a regular sleep schedule would act as another nonmedicinal aid to alleviate pain. One should establish a routine of winding-down activities and go to bed at the same time every night. One should never take naps in the daytime, as this would hamper sleeping through the night. Jude and I had found this "no naps" policy impossible to follow. The day she left the hospital, I found a note from her on my bed which read simply: "Whatever they say, I still think that naps are great!" I too have found that without that midafternoon downtime, I am completely dysfunctional by nightfall. This daily need to take to my bed, I know, has a touch of Victorian melodrama to it; nevertheless, I have come to rely on the sheer pleasure of cozying into my bed midafternoon with my perfect osteopedic pillow and my huge down comforter.

So, there we have the empirical problem: two conflicting opinions, each offering disparate advice, indeed, oppositional advice: Hot compresses or cold? Naps or no naps? Whom to trust? Where to turn for the correct answer? To the Chinese herbalist, osteopath, anesthesiologist, holistic masseuse, kinesthesiologist, Buddhist guru, craniosacral specialist, acupuncturist, or yet another neurosurgeon? The honest truth is that I have learned to trust only myself—ultimately, for all of the doctors' advice, I know my body best and what helps it. This self-assurance had taken more than a year to acquire, as it goes against our society's assumption that a doctor is the accepted expert, and for so long, it felt too perilous to ignore the wisdom of medical science. I have come to realize that my body is mercurial, mysterious, elusive. I can barely understand its shifts and symptoms. To expect a doctor who has only my hospital records and X-rays to understand my body better than I do is unrealistic.

I have also found that educating myself further dispels many of the fears and uncertainties that gripped me in the first year a.p. I have learned about the latest and most promising advances in the field of pain management as well as much more about the diagnosis and treatment of my condition. Books, articles in scientific journals, even the Internet, have all been welcome sources of information, to a great extent demystifying what had felt a year ago like an out-of-control chain of events. Instead of remaining infantilized, allowing doctors to tell me what to do or ingest without clearly understanding why or the risks, I have begun to research these issues for myself. Being the well-educated consumer of medical care gives me back a semblance of agency and control so sorely lacking in the first year of chronic pain. I have also realized that taking control of my physical health, even to the point of being aggressive at doctor's appointments about what I need by way of medication, injections, and psychological help, has proven not only self-empowering but also critical to receiving better care than I used to receive.

CHAPTER 37

Grounded

And it occurs to me that what is crucial is to believe
in effort, to believe some good will come of simply trying
. . . What are we without this?
Whirling in the dark universe,
alone, afraid, unable to influence fate—
　　—LOUISE GLÜCK, from "The Empty Glass"

～～ My mother's friend Barbara had given me the advice early on to act like I felt good and at some point, maybe I would. In other words, I needed to change not only my thoughts but also my actions. Barbara turned out to be right. By behaving less like I am on my deathbed, I have found that I feel less like I am. I even find at times that by acting healthy, I can forget about the pain.

Ironically, this realization came only after further injuring myself. In my efforts to become strong and hardy, I managed to fall while exercising and broke my wrist. Again, the original wrist fracture sustained in the car accident had not held up over time, and what would have been a fairly benign fall for most people led to a shattered wrist for me. This fall set off a huge physical and mental reaction; it acted as a corrective, forcing me to reevaluate, yet again, how I was living my life.

In my second winter a.p., endorphins had become my newest form of methadone. I had swung from one extreme—bedridden patient—to another, superjock ballerina. Only a few short months after first getting out of bed, I found myself in perpetual motion, spending whole afternoons at dance classes, pushing myself as hard as any professional dancer. During those hours, I was blissfully unaware of myself as wrecked, a John Chamberlain sculpture of a body; rather I was Anna Pavlova, pushing myself to achieve new private goals. After class, floating from the rush, I felt compelled to keep moving, to keep the rush going, and so would walk home. The problem was that I couldn't stop. I became dimly aware that when I stopped, I was forced to look inward again and would refocus on my physical problems. Pain, which had been hovering right below the surface, would rush to the fore, and I would morph back into the startled, distorted woman staring at her reflection in a fun-house mirror. This period of running from myself was of course destined to crash, which it appropriately did while in motion.

My family promptly "grounded" me. No leaping. No skiing. No running. No skating. No flying. "You are not allowed to fall and break anything today, OK?" Jackie would joke with me. I have come to agree with my family. My body is ridiculous in its propensity for breaking. So while I might desperately want to be "normal," I know I never will be. And even though I am again functional and have an absurdly high tolerance for pain, my body will always be more fragile than that of the normal person. While ballet remains my daily medicine, I no longer push myself so hard or so far, choosing instead moderation, that middle road that tempers experience and expectation.

Breaking my wrist also forced me to examine how I interacted with the people in my life. I finally put a moratorium on harnessing and receiving excessive amounts of familial attention for my physical problems. The moment the accident happened, I knew it was serious. My forearm looked like a fork, and my hand was dangling off of my wrist. I called Jackie from the emergency room, the only person I felt I could trust with this latest stupidity. My parents were in town, and I thought that if I called them or Eric, I would set them over the edge. (This instinct was, by the way, accurate.)

When the doctor advised surgery, I had a bit of a breakdown. I kept insisting that I couldn't go through another surgery. The pain was also intense enough that I found myself imploring Jackie, "How am I going to do this? I can't handle any more pain." Jackie, one of the most empathetic people I know, remained calm. She ushered me through the ordeal, allowed me to squeeze her hand, whimper, and cry while the doctor set my arm, and then proceeded to babysit me at her apartment for four days before and after the surgery. In those few days, I managed to put a hole in her poncho, break her computer, and order her about so incessantly that she briefly cracked. Mortified, I retreated to my parents' apartment. I had been obliged to confess the accident to my mother once surgery was involved. She was still in town, and there was no way to hide this latest absurdity from her. She had hit the breaking point with me by now as well. Every time I asked her to do something for me, she would mutter under her breath, "I'm just a servant of the realm. A servant of the realm, I tell you. I do as I'm told." Within a few hours, I had overstayed my welcome there, too, and had to skulk back to my sister's apartment. After another day of shuttling between their apartments, I went home to Brooklyn with a new attitude.

I have taken off my tiara and fired the servants. I no longer need or want everyone to rally constantly, incessantly, around me or treat our family as one in crisis. My family had spent the prior year in a constant state of worry about me, and the bedside vigil had infiltrated every moment of our lives. Me, center stage, victim-cripple-invalid moaning, the recipient of an overflow of emotional support and material comforts: flowers, letters, books, tapes, CDs, food, and clothing. I had burdened everyone in my family long enough. I have finally let my sisters off the hook; they are no longer obliged to play nursemaids every weekend. There are no more gratuitous visits to Brooklyn; I meet my sisters or parents in Manhattan somewhere fun—a museum, store, restaurant, hair salon, or theater. Phone calls no longer revolve around my latest symptoms or doctors' visits. I also don't rely on my mother to swoop in and rescue us; I handle our domestic lives—with help, to be sure, from Eric or someone I pay; never-theless, I feel more competent by reclaiming this area of respon-sibility.

In my social interactions, in general, I have learned to practice independence. I generally shrug off the inevitable questions about my health nowadays or simply reveal the truth dispassion-ately. I try to behave with some reticence about my daily pain levels, treatments, and problems. If I am having a difficult pain day, I will admit to it if questioned, but not belabor the discus-sion; and I refuse to divulge such details unless asked. My new approach is to spare people, to shield them from the concern and fear that accompanies knowing the reality.

I am equally matter-of-fact with my close friends. I had over-burdened my intimate friends the first year a.p., causing them to worry inordinately about me. Although I would say that we shouldn't discuss my status, I would routinely bawl on the phone and frequently detail with far too much specificity the latest is-sues in my diagnosis and treatment. My new approach in the second year was to fly in precisely the opposite direction and avoid my inner circle during a spike. I stopped answering my phone and buried myself in order to avoid people, but I found that those who care about me want to know how I am doing. As Lisa said in the midst of a weeklong spike when I could no lon-ger evade her phone calls, "I refuse to let you disappear." She then threatened to hound me even more aggressively if I went under again. Admitting to those I trust that I am having a diffi-cult time often dispels the loneliness and desperation I still feel during rougher pain days.

I have come to rely on this support. At Jackie's apartment a few hours after I broke my wrist, I called home to tell Lilly and Benjamin the news. A mere thirteen minutes later, Lisa called to offer comfort. Lilly had told her friend Daisy about my accident who had told her mother Amanda who had told Lisa. The other line began beeping, thirteen minutes and some seconds later. It was Susan. Benjamin had told his friend Nico who had told his sister Nina who had told her mother Leslie who had told Susan. I joked with Benjamin, just entering the treacherous teenage years. "Benj, thirteen minutes—that's all the time I will ever need to know when you have done something wrong. Guaranteed, whether I want to know or not." Thirteen minutes. That's all the time needed for relevant news to spread, for mothers to mobilize, for aid to be offered.

The past two years have been a process of natural selection; only the most hardy friendships have survived. So, too, as Darwin would have predicted, these friendships have evolved. By bearing witness to so much of my anguish, my friends have become more intimate with me. In the second year, I became aware of just how reciprocal these alliances had become. I would receive a call from a friend on whom I had leaned heavily in the first year; she would admit, "I really need you right now," and then divulge private matters, ones, I think, she would not have felt as safe disclosing prior to my crisis. Friends whom I had taken for granted and only made the effort to see haphazardly have again become an important part of Eric's and my daily lives. Remembering how to be a good friend has helped pull me out of my former self-centeredness and dysphoria.

Having an intimate exchange with a friend or family member thrusts me into my present, and one needs presence for the present. By becoming absorbed by and even in the moment, I have found that my pain recedes. The conversation provides a privileged space in which to get lost, one not replicated in one's exchanges with children, bosses, subordinates (or, in my case, students), or acquaintances. It also doesn't require the intellectual rigor of my work conversations. If I have a bad case of aphasia, then we laugh about it, my friend or mother suggesting words sometimes apt, sometimes so ludicrous that they lead to more glee.

Having fun with friends has become a privileged pain management strategy. Sometimes a raucous belly laugh, a fit of hysterical cackles, a bit of wildness does the most to offset a pain spike. I sat at dinner recently with Benjamin; two of his surf instructors, Java and Sunshine; Holly; and her daughter Chloe. Chloe and Benjamin were wearing three-foot-wide sombreros, giggling at every silly thing that Sunshine said. When he began teasing Holly about how insane her hair looked, I laughed harder and louder than I had in almost two years. Guffawing, I felt my head ache; guffawing louder, I chose to ignore it.

I also seek out daily adventure and look for opportunities that will pull me outside of my known and predictable daily routine—for example, going with a friend to a sculpture park, museum, or neighborhood to which I have never been before. I now walk across the Brooklyn Bridge or in unknown neighborhoods nearly daily with friends. Visits to Bay Ridge to see the Christmas decorations on the houses, to the Brooklyn Botanic Garden to see the cherry blossoms, or to Coney Island to walk on the beach offer breaths of the new and hint at further soon-to-be-discovered joys. These adventures and the process of search and discovery—whether of a friend's emotional state or of a new neighborhood—so fully engage and absorb my mind and emotions that I find myself both acting and feeling like I am in less pain. Barbara's behavioral approach to pain—that is, act like it's not there and maybe it won't be—has proved beautifully apt.

CHAPTER 38

The Fall into Joy

What else to say?
We end in joy.
　　—THEODORE ROETHKE, from "The Moment"

To harness joy is to tame a wild cat: it can't be done. A moment, an hour, is all one should aspire to achieve. Yet during the first year a.p., I had lost the capacity for even such "moments of being." A friend had asked me after my return from the hospital, "But don't you ever feel joy anymore?" She meant the kind of buzzy, synesthetic joy when the senses leap out of their vehicles. One smells with one's eyes; one hears with one's tongue; and the body becomes one. A tuning fork capable of only one pitch, I had lost the ability to feel on such multiple levels. Pain had leveled me, flattening my senses to a lukewarm gray.

Joy has again become available. At times, it is a more ephemeral, less embodied form of joy. Not epiphanic, it has a slow warmth, a glow about it, a warm cup of tea on a winter's day, soft silk against the skin, a low chuckle with my best friend. Perhaps "contentment" would be the more appropriate word. No cup runneth over here. The cup is half full. This more subdued joy, nevertheless, has the potential to outlive the momentary joy: it has also begun to provide me with a way of life, a way back to feeling something more than just pain and effort and obligation.

In the second spring a.p., I had felt such a gaping hole. Hungry, I was so life-hungry. I began to see that only a new fall, this time into such joy, could diminish the consequences of my original fall. I had learned a great deal at the hospital; I had not yet figured out a way to survive not just for the sake of my family but also for me. I learned how in the second year of pain, and it led me back to myself.

One of the methods taught at the clinic for riding out the inevitable pain spikes is "diversion." One should distract oneself with simple, pleasurable activities that take one's mind far away rather than simply lying helpless in bed, aware of every minute pain path. Any number of activities works to bring about such distraction. I found to my surprise that knitting and making jewelry were popular diversions with chronic pain sufferers. In one of my first classes at the clinic, I noticed three other patients busily knitting. I realized that I had somehow found a way of self-medicating in those long hours deep in the winter nights. Other distractions popular with patients at the hospital included playing card games, cooking, and gardening.

I came to associate these diversionary tactics, however, with the comatose stagnation and inertia that my life had become in the first years. These activities were simply the means by which I whiled away the hours still with no real purpose or structure. I needed not distractions (or glorified hobbies) but the return of fulfillment and passion. My family had at various times in the first year of pain turned to me and said, "You really should write about your experience." I had been in no condition that year to read, let alone write, a book; and I would respond sometimes bitterly, more often in despair: "Sometimes it's just the sheer enduring that is the achievement." Wasn't that self-evident? Abashed, my family was confronted with such a transformed philosophy that they often had no response. Surrounded by so many overachieving, ambitious, well-educated individuals, I knew that the refusal (or inability) to turn one's life opportunities and experiences into some kind of professional achievement or creative fodder was an anathema. And, for my midwestern parents, in particular, who wanted their daughters to transcend their roots, be extraordinary, and live big lives, my experience needed to end triumphantly. There would be a cure for my pain; moreover, I would have a book about the experience to show for it. Of course, my experience would have a nice, clean, linear structure, and the genre would undoubtedly be comedy—that is, regardless of the missteps, misunderstandings, and confusions early in the plotline, it would necessarily have a happy ending. Such a book I cannot write.

This book thus began as an act of defiance, perhaps competing with the book everyone hoped that I would write. My inspiration for this book arose, however, not from internal compulsion at first, but from the suggestion of my friend Sue. While listening to me discuss my experiences, she had commented, "You have a story to tell, one that could really help others like yourself." I remembered how important it was to bond with other patients at the hospital and thought that many chronic pain sufferers probably don't have a network of friends in a similar situation. They might experience the kind of loneliness and isolation that I had felt during those long winter months. Sue's suggestion sparked something in me, something more palliative than any of my earlier diversions.

She followed up our conversation by sending me Bob and Lee Woodruff's memoir, *In an Instant: A Family's Journey of Love and Healing.* I read it in two days. This marked a significant moment. It was practically the first book I had managed to read in more than a year. Although my pain levels remained high, I found that I could concentrate. I realized only then how much the various opioid narcotics—not the pain itself—had stripped my mind of cognitive ability.

The Woodruffs' survival story, particularly how Bob Woodruff learned to cope with a disabling injury, resonated with me. After gulping down the book, however, I still had issues, questions, unresolved anxieties circulating. I wasn't sure yet how to work through these emotions, but somehow, I gravitated to my fifteen-year-old, antiquated computer, finding its loud hum and dusty keyboard in all its clicky, sticky wobbliness welcoming and familiar. For the first time in well over a year, I began to write again. This was certainly not one of those famous literary epiphanies—Wordsworth on top of Mount Snowdon, James Joyce staring at the bird-girl, Proust tasting that first madeleine—but it somehow distracted me from my constant pain. Without a voice, without the written word, I had spent the year in free fall.

The act of creation competes in a deadly struggle with pain. To create is to dislodge pain from the center, to prioritize and privilege the mind over the body. Creativity also requires an act of will on the part of the pain sufferer. I have learned that I must push myself actively, consciously, to find and appreciate beauty and aesthetic pleasures when in pain. Reaccessing a passion critical to one's soul and spirit, I think, can shore one up better than any distraction.

The disassociated state into which one enters when creating or engaging a true passion, in particular, has worked better for me than the relaxation and meditation exercises as well. For the "obsessive" mind, I think, attempting to engender no-thought or just experiencing the moment through one's breath is a difficult—if not a counterintuitive—activity. Better than trying to empty the mind, I find it both more natural and more healing to exercise, chew on, work over, remake the obsessions into something new. While I have not jettisoned meditation (particularly during a spike), I spend greater parts of my days reading and writing. One friend at the hospital described how playing his drums is an integral part of his life, diametrically at odds with the phonosensitivity he experiences as a migraine patient. He, nevertheless, refuses to give up this passion—even finding that playing helps him to overcome his pain.

There are still those passions that are no longer available: I am too well aware of this. So one must think hard about which passions are still accessible. I also believe what Juju pointed out to me not so long ago: "Passions are transferable." One can transform a passion into a slightly different, more accessible form.

One woman at the hospital had already figured out this important lesson before she arrived. She had originally trained and worked as a family therapist in private practice. When her health problems made this work no longer viable for her, she had turned her interests into an online counseling service. This work has proven fulfilling for her and also realistic, given her pain levels. She can read and answer e-mails on her own time and at her discretion.

I, too, have rethought my passions in order to find ways of making them still feasible, even if in somewhat altered forms. I have been particularly focused on salvaging as much of my former life as possible. Returning to writing as my principal occupation, albeit radically different in its content from my former scholarly writing, was the first step in reconstructing my intellectual life. I have also returned to the simple daily act of reading, although I have not returned to reading—or writing—literary criticism, which still feels daunting, and I wonder whether my mind will ever again find it so fulfilling. Of late, I mostly read contemporary poetry, as I can digest and focus on compact poetry more easily than on longer works. I still refuse to rush into permanent decisions about my working life, and my teaching career remains on hold. I fluctuate between thinking that my current pain levels make teaching unrealistic and that, as my coping skills continue to improve, perhaps I will be able to do my job again.

My biggest priority has been to refind my family and my joy in and for them. When I first got out of the hospital, my initial concern had been to pull our family out of the state of disarray in which it had found itself after the first year. I had accomplished this goal slowly, initially needing to pace myself just to participate part-time in their lives. It wasn't until I got out of bed in November that I became wholly present and reinstated in their daily routines. I had drifted so far from their interests and concerns that I have found that just the simple act of watching

Benjamin's skateboarding tricks, doing homework with Lilly, or eating dinner with them has repaired some of the lost connections.

So, too, going out with my husband again—for dinner, a party, or really any outing when it is just the two of us—has helped us as a couple. For months our relationship revolved around him taking care of me, and we have had to work consciously to reclaim our former intimacy. He remains the calm and compassionate man whom I met twenty-two years ago, one who, I think, is still hoping for me to return to the woman I was. Our feelings for each other have somehow survived.

Reaccessing my own passion for my children and husband remained a tricky business even after I had gotten out of bed, however, as I initially felt like I was going through the motions, putting the effort into connecting for their sakes rather than for my own. I had felt that my obligation and debt to them required my commitment and engagement, so I returned to them for them, rather than for me. It wasn't that I no longer wanted them; it was that I had become so possessed by pain that I didn't really have enough room in me to focus on anything but having the pain exorcised.

This feeling remains a present concern, and pain continues to isolate me in my own self-involvement. The most absorbing relationship of my life, unfortunate to admit, is still pain; it demands too much of me—time, attention, and sheer grit—for this to be otherwise. So it has been a process to learn how to ignore it enough to be able to place my energy and passion back into my family, my friends, work, and other interests. Ultimately, I have found that all of my strategies are simply efforts to ignore this ever-present, omnipotent foe. None of the methods ever cures me. Rather, the techniques make it easier for me to coexist with pain and to feel at least at times comfortable enough in my own skin to be able to look outside of it.

I, therefore, remain focused on approaching the psychological aspects of my life in less destructive ways than I had in the first year a.p. In a recent conversation, the pain doctor opened up a new approach to internalizing my condition. I admitted to continuing feelings of despair, particularly strong during my spikes. He responded by stressing that his philosophy about pain is that one should never give up. One should try any and all means available to cope with ongoing pain and not simply resign oneself to it. Chronic pain is a disease, one that causes ancillary and serious problems to the body: it therefore cannot be simply borne. If he ran out of options, then I should find another doctor with "more tricks up his sleeve." Working aggressively to rid myself of pain, I should rely on both medicinal and nonmedicinal approaches in my daily life.

Practically speaking, this means that I will continue to put my faith in those doctors who have committed themselves to helping me and whom I trust—namely, my neurologists, pain anesthesiologist, and psychologist. I continue to look to them to help me chip away at the pain as well as they can with medications, further procedures (within limits), and psychological buoying.

I have also rethought my former approaches to pain analgesics. As spikes continued to horrify, I began to think it masochistic to suffer needlessly through them; now, during an intense spike, I will at times turn to medication. I am fully versed in the risks of becoming physically dependent upon narcotics again and am rigorous about my usage. I do not take these pills more than two times a week and only take them when the pain is ruthless. This more balanced approach has allowed me greater periods, if not of functionality, then of peace.

Most effectively, I continue to practice nonmedicinal approaches to combat my pain. My primary methods of pain management remain relaxation exercises, pacing myself, taking control of my care, educating myself as to my condition, endorphin rushes, exercise, physical therapy, massage, adequate sleep, distractions, friendships, reading, and writing. I have also found that I must be flexible, as an action that worked last month may not work the following. Conversely, sometimes solutions that had failed in prior months prove ameliorative later.

Even with nonmedicinal approaches to combating pain, I have put down limits. I unceremoniously rejected my mother's surprise introduction of a self-proclaimed healer at a family party. For my mother's sake, I did allow her to embrace me at the party. (The only change I felt was in mood, as I stifled giggles provoked by my uncle Sandy's sardonic grins and raised eyebrows.) I have, however, refused to see this healer for subsequent healing sessions. I have also rejected a list of quackeries, ranging from magnets to large rubber bands wrapped around my head. I appreciate advice, always offered by the well-meaning, but no longer solicit it and gauge for myself how reliable or analgesic such methods sound before rushing out on the next wild-goose chase. It isn't that I rule out or refuse to try new options, but I have learned to proceed with a certain amount of delicacy and caution.

I have mostly found that I have to surround myself with a coterie of armed archangels who help me fight off Satan, swapping and trading off all of my weapons, medicinal and non-medical, for battling pain. Some days, I wield endorphins; other days, I parry with a narcotic; sometimes I practice stealth and escape into a three-hour nap; and at other times, I try detonating my enemy with a new injection.

My life in some ways resembles a never-ending battle; in other ways, it resembles a circus, garish, dizzying, off-kilter. An underbelly of violence threatens to topple the tent at any time. I play the role of a magician, with sleights of hand and tricks up my sleeve, or a juggler, struggling to keep several options afloat, or a tightrope walker, balancing precariously and hoping that I don't fall again. Sometimes, I'm simply a clown, foolish in my efforts; other times, I'm a lion tamer, wielding a whip, trying to wrestle pain into control before it whips me. I have mostly learned that it is a three-ring circus—not a one-man show. All the other people in my life are as affected by my pain as I, and they demand center stage, too. Lately, I am most happy when I can become just a side act and defer to Eric, Benjamin, or Lilly to play the lead.

Recently Eric and I attended the spring dance concert at my children's school. We held hands, surrounded by close friends, as we watched both Lilly and Benjamin perform that evening. African drums beat louder and faster as the evening progressed, and the stage vibrated with the power of the children's bodies. Lilly swirled in gray chiffon, looking tall and composed as ever, her face set in earnest concentration. Then Benjamin danced his solo; he was a blur of motion, long and loose limbed, his movements subtle and precise. Uninhibited, he gave himself over to the rhythm as cheers broke out. Eric whispered to me, "Look, there are your genes up there," and I fell once more, this time into joy.

CHAPTER 39

Down the Cliff

In either hand the hastening Angel caught
Our lingering parents, and to the eastern gate
Led them direct, and down the cliff as fast
To the subjected plain; then disappeared.
They, looking back, all the eastern side beheld
Of Paradise, so late their happy seat . . .
Some natural tears they dropped, but wiped them soon;
The World was all before them, where to choose
Their place of rest, and Providence their guide:
They, hand in hand, with wandering steps and slow,
Through Eden *took their solitary way.*
    —JOHN MILTON, from *Paradise Lost*

    I find these final lines of *Paradise Lost* so affecting for their balance and harmony, as the human condition—encompassing both tragedy and comedy, despair and desire, grief and solace, hope and resignation—hangs together in perfect equanimity. The Archangel Michael exiles Adam and Eve from Eden, "send[ing] them forth, though sorrowing, yet in peace." They cry but soon wipe their tears away. They depart paradise, "down the cliff," but they begin a journey to a new life, one that God has assured them will at the end of time be providential. They begin their new life alone, taking their "solitary way"; yet, they also leave "hand in hand," acknowledging that while we journey through life alone, we also have a basic human need for contact, intimacy, love, community.

    Like Adam and Eve at the end of the poem, I would be lying if I didn't admit to grief for my old life. I try not to dwell on my life before the onset of pain—lingering in my own paradise lost is painful. I find myself still missing it, and its memories still awaken newly rancorous wounds. I would also be lying if I didn't equally confirm that I have found much to temper these feelings through all of the seismic shifts in my perception on this continuing journey. My life now feels in better equipoise.

The pain spikes, particularly when they go on for several days, still bring me close to an emotional cliff. I still worry over my career, find parenting—properly—a challenge, and experience difficulties behaving as a wife, sister, daughter, colleague, and friend should. I wish I could offer a little recipe for living with chronic pain: a dash of patience, a dollop of faith, mix in some hope and a whole lot of endorphins, perhaps, and voilà, you, too, can survive intact. I also wish that I could follow such a recipe myself, instead of stuttering my way through this life. After having met so many others who suffer from chronic pain, I can say that we all concoct our own unique recipes and then find ourselves needing to rethink and remix the ingredients only a few months later. We share battles with self-doubt, loneliness, self-esteem, worries over the future, our families, and our careers, and sometimes sheer desperation. Our emotional fluctuations are extreme, as we face hourly cliffs and mountains, tidal waves and whirlpools. I crave a day when I don't have to struggle so intensely just to get through it. I also wish that I could declare otherwise.

I have, nevertheless, moved far from the fallen state in which I found myself that first winter: while not having attained my lost paradise at this point, I do find my feet firmly planted on this fallen earth. And, as Serena often says: "You must be grounded in order to float."

As Adam and Eve depart paradise, they begin a journey with a still unknown destination. We are all works in progress, and the process of reinvention for every human being, not just pain sufferers, is endless. My journey, even in its latest incarnation, has not yet landed me anywhere. I veer off the road and investigate new trails. Other times, I run headlong down a hill and trip. Occasionally, I still find myself getting lost. Sometimes, I simply stretch out along a path and look up at the sky. I continue to move forward, nonetheless, learning better ways of coping with my pain, still not certain of my final destination, or of whether this pain will improve, and, if so, by how much. I balance this uncertainty with the will to work proactively to improve my daily life. Most days, I refuse to let the pain defeat me; on the days when it does, I try for the simple comforts: a warm bed, an apt book of poetry (usually elegies, I admit), and chocolate.

A frustrating but nevertheless realistic truism is that all chronic pain sufferers must learn to compensate for the limits demanded of us by our bodies and work hard to attain some quality of life. I have learned that this burden is lightened not by simply being stalwart, bearing the inevitable setbacks, but by clinging to hope, even if guardedly, cautiously, for some respite from the ongoing pain. Medical advances are made every day, and the study of neurology continues to be a growing field. I stay in the realm of realism but always carry with me the fantasy, the romance, the wish fulfillment—the poetry of hope.

Author's Note

⟨᷐᷐⟩ One in every five adult Americans lives with chronic pain (pain that lasts for several months)—from cancer, fibromyalgia, headaches, back problems, rheumatoid arthritis, osteoarthritis, lupus, multiple sclerosis, or neuralgia, to name just a few of the causes. Approximately 45 million Americans alone live with persistent neck pain and headaches. *Newsweek* magazine in a June 2007 cover story reported: "Chronic pain is one of the most pervasive and intractable medical conditions in the United States." Understood as a disease, chronic pain has no clear cure or treatment. *The New York Times Magazine* in a June 2007 cover story noted that "[c]ontrary to the old saw, pain kills. A body in pain produces high levels of hormones that cause stress to the heart and lungs. Pain can cause blood pressure to spike, leading to heart attacks and strokes. Pain can also consume so much of the body's energy that the immune system degrades." *The New York Times* in a subsequent article in "Health News" suggested that even after significant pain management intervention, only about 50 percent of the afflicted are able to resume their jobs. As *Newsweek* quite sensitively pointed out, pain has sometimes catastrophic effects on the lives of many sufferers: "The cascade of changes in the nervous system can lead to an equally painful cascade of events in a patient's life: memory loss, job loss, marital strife, depression, suicide."

My story, then, is not unique. Pain derailed me, like millions of others, insinuating itself into a happy life. My family, watching helplessly in the wake of pain's onslaught, found themselves hurting, too. I dedicate this book to people in chronic pain and to those who love and care for them. For you who have found your lives similarly wrenched, even irrecoverably lost, I hope that you will each find that mysterious, personal combination of methods that will help you to rebuild your lives with new goals and meaning while still retaining some essence of your old selves.

Appendix *Selected Poetry*

⟿ One of the mechanisms I have to cope with chronic pain is poetry. No longer a critic, but rather an appreciator, I have found that many of my favorite poets have grappled with their own pain—psychic, emotional, and sometimes physical. They have described this pain in ways that resonate deeply with my own reality. Short lyric bursts of poetry in particular offer words of comfort, consolation, and camaraderie. I offer here a few of the poems that have most moved me and given order, form, and meaning to my experience.

I Felt a Funeral in My Brain

I felt a Funeral, in my Brain,
And Mourners to and fro
Keep treading—treading—till it seemed
That Sense was breaking through—

And when they all were seated,
A service, like a Drum—
Kept beating—beating—till I thought
My Mind was going numb—

And then I heard them lift a Box
And creak across my Soul
With those same Boots of Lead, again,
Then Space—began to toll,

As all the Heavens were a Bell,
And Being, but an Ear,
And I, and Silence, some strange Race
Wrecked, solitary, here—

And then a Plank in Reason, broke,
And I dropped down, and down—
And hit a World, at every plunge,
And Finished knowing—then—

—Emily Dickinson

Brief Reflections on the Word "Pain"

Wittgenstein says: the words "It hurts" have replaced
    tears and cries of pain. The word "Pain"
    does not describe the expression of pain but
            replaces it.
    Thus it creates a new behaviour pattern
    in the case of pain.

The word enters between us and the pain
    like a pretence of silence.
    It is a silencing. It is a needle
    unpicking the stitch
    between blood and clay.

The word is the first small step
    to freedom
    from oneself.

In case others
    are present.

—Miroslav Holub

From *Contradictions: Tracking Poems* (Section 7)

Dear Adrienne,
                    I feel signified by pain
from my breastbone through my left shoulder down
through my elbow into my wrist is a thread of pain
I am typing this instead of writing by hand

because my wrist on the right side
blooms and rushes with pain
like a neon bulb
You ask me how I'm going to live
the rest of my life
Well, nothing is predictable with pain
Did the old poets write of this?
—in its odd spaces, free,
many have sung and battled—
But I'm already living the rest of my life
not under conditions of my choosing
wired   into pain
                              rider on the slow train
                                        Yours, Adrienne

—Adrienne Rich

HEAD-ACH.
(Written in her fifteenth year, 1829)

Head-ach! thou bane to Pleasure's fairy spell,
Thou fiend, thou foe to joy, I know thee well!
Beneath thy lash I've writhed for many an hour,—
I hate thee, for I've known, and dread thy power.

Even the heathen gods were made to feel
The aching torments which thy hand can deal;
And Jove, the ideal king of heaven and earth,
Owned thy dread power, which called stern Wisdom forth.

Wouldst thou thus ever bless each aching head,
And bid Minerva make the brain her bed,
Blessings might then be taught to rise from woe,
And Wisdom spring from every throbbing brow.

But always the reverse to me, unkind,
Folly for ever dogs thee close behind;

And from this burning brow, her cap and bell,
For ever jingle Wisdom's funeral knell.

—Lucretia Maria Davidson

First Poem After Serious Surgery

The breath continues but the breathing
hurts
Is this the way death wins its way
against all longing
and redemptive thrust from grief?
Head falls
Hands crawl
and pain becomes the only keeper
of my time

I am not held
I do not hold
And touch degenerates into new
agony

I feel
the healing of cut muscle/
broken nerves
as I return to hot and cold
sensations
of a body tortured by the flight
of feeling/normal
registrations of repulsion
or delight

On this meridian of failure or recovery
I move
or stop respectful
of each day

but silent now
and slow

—June Jordan

The Recovery Zone

If I could befriend this pain,
could consider the wracking
of the spirit
a kind of exercise,

if I could see myself
in pure perspective: no more
than a comma in the long epic
of suffering,

then I would slake my thirst
with these salty tears
and decorate my pale body
with love's bloody stigmata.

—Linda Pastan

Resurrection of the Right Side

When the half-body dies its frightful death
forked pain, infection of snakes, lightning, pull down
    the voice.   Waking
and I begin to climb the mountain on my mouth,
word by stammer, walk stammered, the lurching deck of
    earth.
Left-right with none of my own rhythms
the long-established sex and poetry.
                                        I go running in sleep,
but waking stumble down corridors of self, all rhythms
    gone.

The broken movement of love   sex out of rhythm
one halted name   in a shattered language
ruin of French-blue lights behind the eyes
slowly the left hand extends a hundred feet
and the right hand follows follows
but still the power of sight is very weak
but I go rolling this ball of life, it rolls
and I follow it whole up the slowly-brightening slope

A whisper attempts me, I whisper without stammer
I walk the long hall to the time of a metronome
set by a child's gun-target   left-right
the power of eyesight is very slowly arriving
   in this late impossible daybreak
   all the blue flowers open

—Muriel Rukeyser

The Body Mutinies
—outside Saint Pete's

When the doctor runs out of words and still
I won't leave, he latches my shoulder and
steers me out doors. Where I see his blurred hand,
through the milk glass, flapping goodbye like a sail
(& me not griefstruck yet but still amazed: how
words and names—medicine's blunt instruments—
undid me. And the seconds, the half seconds
it took for him to say those words.) For now,
I'll just stand in the courtyard, watching bodies
struggle in then out of one lean shadow
a tall fir lays across the wet flagstones,
before the sun clears the valance of gray trees
and finds the surgical-supply shop window
and makes the dusty bedpans glint like coins.

—Lucia Perillo

The Parasite

The doctor looked angry
and I too began to choke
with rage at those shadows
who take up all our time
with their uncontrollable desire.

The doctor removed his glasses
and began to clean them
pensively with the hem of his gown.
The room became hazy, intimate.
A file cabinet hovered beside me.
The doctor was a small white cloud.

At once I saw clearly:
it was all my fault.
The bitterness, dizziness
in middle age, a fall,
the beautiful work
suddenly turned incoherent.

The doctor put his fingers together
as if they fitted a special way—
a gesture that would take years to master
and there was so little time,
every second was measured—

and he spoke very softly.
I sensed his great weariness.
I wanted to rock him in my arms.
Rest, he said, night after night
of sleep without terrible dreams.
And work. And loved ones.
Patience, said the doctor, barely audible
above the sweet constant music.

—D. Nurkse

Sonnet 21

Sing the gardens, my heart, that you do not know; like
    gardens
poured in glass, clear, unattainable.
Waters and roses of Ispahan or of Shiraz,
blissfully sing them, praise them, comparable to none.

Show, my heart, that you never miss them. That it is
you they have in mind, their ripening figs.
That you consort with their airs that are heightened
as though to vision between the blossoming branches.

Avoid the error of thinking something is missed
for the resolve once taken, this: to be!
Silken thread, you became part of the weaving,

Whichever the picture you are innerly one with
(be it even a moment out of the life of pain),
feel that the whole, the glorious carpet is meant.

—Rainer Maria Rilke

Acknowledgments

To each and every member of my extended family who buoyed, and continues to buoy, me, particularly my husband, Eric; my children, Benjamin and Lilly; my parents, Jan and Ronald Greenberg; my sisters, Jeanne Greenberg Rohatyn and Jackie Greenberg; brother-in-law Nicolas Rohatyn; parents-in-law Mike and Maria Avram; and brothers- and sisters-in-law Jonny Shaman, Rella and Joe Hartman, Marc and Robin Avram, Mathew and Alison Avram, and David and Kristy Avram. Sincere thanks as well to cousins Andrew and Lisa Blatt, Chris and Kristen Viela, Lilly Schonwald, Lee Newman, and Betsy Cohen, Uncle Sandy Schonwald, and Uncle Bob and Aunt Maureen Greenberg. My deepest gratitude to Maria Corazon Resurreccion, Georgina Cerf, and Amparo Espinosa.

To coffee girls Lisa Zabel, Susan Bruce, Amanda Moffat, and Leslie Marshall, and their husbands, Richard Zabel, Peter Hedges, Jimmy Moffat, and Mauro Premutico. To best friends Audrey Stone, Tamir Rosenblum, Jillisa Brittan, Susannah Blinkoff, and Betsy Schechter. To girls' night girls Holly Peterson, hub and best friend to us all; Juju Chang; Heather Vincent; Andrea Wong; Amy Rosenberg; Jody Friedman; Betsy West; Dabber Wentworth; and honorary girls' night girls, Rick Kimball and Neal Shapiro. To Joseph Wittreich, my mentor, whom I have never allowed to stop mentoring me, and to my first mentor, Patrick Cullen. To surrogate parents Barbara Messing and Gene Spector, Sally Peterson and Michael Carlisle, and Elaine and Donald Sharpe.

To Hunter colleagues Cristina Alfar, Sarah Chinn, Rebecca Connor, Donna Masini, Thom Taylor, and Michael Thomas and, in addition, to Meena Alexander, Karen Greenberg, Marlene Hennessey, Nico Israel, Jan Heller Levi, Harriet Luria, Nondita Mason, Evelyn Melamed, Mark Miller, Kate Parry, Charles Persky, and Gary Schmidgall for reaching out to me.

To all of Eric's ABC colleagues, especially Mary Kate Burke, Samantha Chapman, Roger Sergel, Dr. Tim Johnson, Kris Sebastian, Mimi Gurbst, Diane Sawyer, Chris Cuomo, and Cynthia McFadden.

To Gabrielle Howard and John Smith, heads of the Lower and Upper Middle Schools of Saint Ann's School, who have so sensitively accommodated our family, and to two particularly important teachers in Lilly's life: Chandra Speeth and Julia Hart.

To Doctors Joel Saper, David Gordan, Shamas Moheyuddin, Rebecca Kotlowski, and Alan Lake, as well as Celeste Fraser, Jeff Osworth, Leslie Cunningham, and Ivy Friess. Heartfelt admiration and gratitude to Jude Proschanski, Jill Penny, Ben Hodges, Susan Hogenson-Boon, Lyn Marx, Moselle Graves, and Dee Botero.

To New York doctors Brenda Berger, Daniel Richman, Deborah Deliyannides, and Sandra Berman. A special thank-you to Serena Schrier and One-on-One Physical Therapy, particularly Jesse Simon.

For those unexpected gestures and acts of kindness that made so much of a difference, I thank Amy Adler, Stephanie Anuszkiewicz, Java Bailey, Megan Barrett, Paula Berry, Claire Bonner, Jody Brandt, Brenda Breslauer, Tim and Meiken Brown, Karen Burnes, Francie Campbell, Nina Collins, Francesca Connelly, Colette Corry, Martha Dietz, Debbie Dingle, Victoria Elenowitz, Barbara Everdell, Jane Garnett and David Booth, Joey Haddad and Michael O'Laughlin, Paul Hurley, Piotr Jagninski, Harold Koplewicz, Mark Larson, Marlene Malek, Barbara Marcus, Sunshine Margaritis, Amy Margolis, Caroline Marshall, Jeanne Messing, James Meyer, Linda Resnick, Jeanette Rohatyn, Michael Rohatyn, Elissa Santissi and Jim Keller, Helene Sayad, Danner Schefler, Mariza Scotch, Laurie Simmons, the Jewish

Center of the Hamptons's cantor Debra Stein and director of education Shelley Lichtenstein, Kristen Steinke, Dick Wyman, Paula Grieff Zanes, and fellow Miltonists Sharon Achinstein, Carol Barton, Rosanna Cox, Stuart Curran, Tony Demarest, Stephen Dobranski, Charles Durham, Richard Durocher, Mimi Fenton, Peter Herman, Jameela Lares, John Leonard, Kris Pruitt, Louis Schwartz, Rachel Trubowitz, Sara Van Den Berg, and Susanne Woods.

To my editor, Susan Mercandetti, who both inspired this book and worked so hard to improve it, and to all at Random House who nurtured this book, especially Abby Plesser, Millicent Bennett, Robbin Schiff, Sally Marvin, Jennifer Huwer, and Steve Messina. And to Adrienne Davich, Lynn Goldberg, and Megan Beattie. Many thanks as well to photographers Nancy Crampton, Ken Schles, and Marilyn Minter.

Finally, a too-long-belated thank-you and indebtedness to Clayton Varley, June Varley, Miriam Tennenbaum, and Peggy Schmidt.

Permission Credits

Hughes. Rights outside of the United States are controlled by Faber and Faber Ltd. Reprinted by permission of HarperCollins Publishers and Faber and Faber Ltd.

HarperCollins Publishers and Jonathan Cape, a member of The Random House Group Ltd.: Excerpt from "Mercy on Broadway" from *Sweet Machine* by Mark Doty, coypright © 1998 by Mark Doty. Rights throughout the British Commonwealth are controlled by Jonathan Cape, a member of The Random House Group Ltd. Reprinted by permission of HarperCollins Publishers and Jonathan Cape, a member of The Random House Group Ltd.

HarperCollins Publishers and Michael Katz: "Nothing Lasts" from *Given Sugar, Given Salt* by Jane Hirshfield, coypright © 2001 by Jane Hirshfield. Rights outside of North America are controlled by Michael Katz. Reprinted by permission of HarperCollins Publishers and Michael Katz.

HarperCollins Publishers and The Wylie Agency LLC: Excerpts from *Howl* by Allen Ginsberg, copyright © 1955 by Allen Ginsberg, copyright © 2006 by The Allen Ginsberg Trust. Rights throughout the British Commonwealth are controlled by The Wylie Agency LLC. Reprinted by permission of HarperCollins Publishers and The Wylie Agency LLC.

Harvard University Press: "I Felt a Funeral in My Brain" from *The Poems of Emily Dickinson* by Emily Dickinson, edited by Thomas H. Johnson (Cambridge, Mass.: The Belknap Press of Harvard University Press), copyright © 1951, 1955, 1979, 1983 by The President and Fellows of Harvard College. Reprinted by permission of the publishers and the Trustees of Amherst College.

Houghton Mifflin Harcourt Publishing Company: Excerpt from "XLV" from *The Triumph of Love* by Geoffrey Hill, copyright © 1998 by Geoffrey Hill. Reprinted by permission of Houghton Mifflin Harcourt Publishing Company.

Houghton Mifflin Harcourt Publishing Company and SLL/Sterling Lord Literistic, Inc.: Excerpt from "The Break" from *Love Poems* by Anne Sexton, copyright © 1967, 1968, 1969 by Anne Sexton. Rights throughout the British Commonwealth are controlled by SLL/

About the Author

LYNNE GREENBERG is an associate professor of English at Hunter College. Her academic writing focuses on seventeenth-century British literature. She has a J.D. from the University of Chicago Law School and a Ph.D. from the City University of New York's Graduate School and University Center. She lives in New York City with her husband and their two children.

About the Type

This book was set in Centaur, a typeface designed by the American typographer Bruce Rogers in 1929. Centaur was a typeface that Rogers adapted from the fifteenth-century type of Nicolas Jenson and modified in 1948 for a cutting by the Monotype Corporation.